The Zoonoses

**Infections
transmitted from animals to man**

Jack Payne died unexpectedly on March 19, 1988 after this manuscript was completed but before publication. We have lost a valued colleague and friend.

JCB
SRP

The Zoonoses

Infections transmitted from animals to man

John C. Bell   BVSc MRCVS DVSM
Senior Veterinary Officer,
Veterinary Investigation Section,
Ministry of Agriculture Fisheries & Food,
Tolworth

Stephen R. Palmer   MA MB BChir FFCM
Consultant Epidemiologist,
PHLS Communicable Disease
Surveillance Centre,
PHLS Regional Epidemiologist for Wales,
Cardiff Public Health Laboratory,
University Hospital of Wales, Cardiff

Jack M. Payne   PhD BSc MRCVS FiBiol
FRSA
Late Visiting Professor,
Department of Agriculture,
University of Reading,
(Formerly Director the ASRC Institute for
Research on Animal Disease, Compton)

Edward Arnold

A division of Hodder & Stoughton

LONDON   BALTIMORE   MELBOURNE   AUCKLAND

© 1988 John C. Bell, Stephen R. Palmer, Jack M. Payne

First published in Great Britain 1988

British Library Cataloguing in Publication Data
Bell, John C.
  The Zoonoses.
  1. Man. Zoonoses
  I. Title II. Palmer, Stephen R.
  III. Payne, Jack M.
  616.9'59
  ISBN 0-7131-4561-7

Typeset in 10/11 pt Times by Colset Private Limited, Singapore.
Printed and bound in Great Britain for Edward Arnold, the
educational, academic and medical publishing division of Hodder
and Stoughton Limited, 41 Bedford Square, London WC1B 3DQ by
Richard Clay Ltd, Suffolk.

Contents

Preface

The idea for a handbook on zoonoses began in 1982. It followed, somewhat circuitously, from a report presented to the Agricultural Working Group appointed by the Committee for Information on Science and Documentation (CIDST) of the Commission of the European Communities in Luxembourg. A Task Force was set up to devise a computerized data bank on zoonoses which initially included information on only 37 zoonoses of top priority. However, in common with many other computerized data banks, it suffered disadvantages. Accessibility was limited to users who not only knew it existed but also possessed an on-line computer terminal. Furthermore the 37 zoonoses represented only a proportion of the total. Thus we prepared a more comprehensive listing in handbook form for general and popular use.

We defined a zoonosis as 'an infectious disease naturally transmissible between vertebrates and man'. This fits the concept of zoonosis as accepted by the World Health Organization. A great variety of such diseases occur. Some have complex cycles of infection involving intermediate hosts, whilst others spread by environmental contamination. Some inflict highly fatal, severe disease (e.g. rabies, anthrax and tuberculosis) whereas others initiate outbreaks of relatively mild, but potentially incapacitating, illness (e.g. salmonellosis and campylobacteriosis).

Zoonoses have emerging importance. In part this arises from increasing public awareness of the danger of infections introduced in foods of animal origin. Thus producers are more and more forced to assure the safety of their products and consumers are better educated on the best ways for storing, handling and cooking of food. In some ways the intensification of animal husbandry worsens the situation by encouraging the spread of infection between animals and by the extra contamination of the environment by the disposal of infected effluent on to pasture or into water-courses. This, coupled with new interest of the urban population in rural leisure pursuits, brings more people into contact with animal diseases. Some, being more venturesome than others, take adventure holidays in foreign parts where exotic disease lurks both in the wildlife and in the local domestic animals. In these circumstances the risks of eating such foods as raw fish, meat or milk must be realized. Similarly such tourists should avoid being bitten by mosquitoes and other biting insects which often carry infection from the wildlife reservoirs of zoonotic disease.

Pets create special problems. Dogs and cats live in close proximity to their owners and transmit disease such as echinococcosis and toxoplasmosis. Even greater dangers are associated with exotic pets such as parrots and monkeys which may harbour potentially fatal infections such as ornithosis and herpes infections. New lifestyles sometimes create special hazards. Both agricultural and urban developments may encroach into previously uncultivated land or forest where new contacts are made with wildlife which may be reservoirs of infections – examples being plague and various types of viral encephalitis. Also, modern trade in agricultural products, wool, skin or hides creates new avenues for the entry of zoonotic disease such as anthrax.

The growing awareness of the problem of zoonosis is such that a world-wide system of specialist centres and public health laboratories now operates to advise and offer diagnostic services. The World Health Organization, based at Geneva, performs a coordination role in this activity. We consider that this handbook has a part to play. We hope it will help guide and warn the public about zoonotic disease and the circumstances in which risks exist. It is especially designed to be read by the veterinary and medical professions because each shares responsibility for preventing zoonoses. We have also tried to set out a simple but comprehensive text, of help to administrators, legislators, planners, tourist operators and others. In particular we realize that progress in the prevention and treatment of zoonotic disease depends on research and the development of new vaccines and chemotherapeutics. Thus the many items in this book labelled simply 'unknown' may provide a spur for future endeavour.

Most of the diseases in this book have been (or still are) known by alternative names. For completeness we have included these in square brackets underneath the main headings.

1988   JCB
                                              SRP
                                              JMP

African trypanosomiasis

[African sleeping sickness, Gambian trypanosomiasis, Rhodesian trypanosomiasis]

A common, chronic, and often fatal protozoal infection of humans in tropical Africa (mainly between latitudes 20°N and 20°S). It is usually transmitted by the tsetse fly and occurs both in outbreaks and sporadically.

The causative agents are *Trypanosoma brucei gambiense* and *T. b. rhodesiense* (Protozoa). There is no vaccine.

Reservoir and mode of transmission
Many wild and domestic animals harbour infection. In Gambian trypanosomiasis, humans are the main reservoir and source of infection for the vector tsetse fly (*Glossina palpalis*, *G. tachinoides* or *G. fuscipes*). The tsetse fly is infected when it bites during the parasitaemic phases and the trypanosome develops in the vector, culminating in infection of its saliva; transmission is by the tsetse fly bite. In Rhodesian trypanosomiasis, animals, especially domestic cattle and pigs, play an important role as reservoirs. In humans, intrauterine infection has been recorded.

Incubation period
Humans. Usually 3–21 days for *T. b. rhodesiense* but longer and highly variable for *T. b. gambiense*.

Animals. Usually subclinical in domestic and wild animals.

Clinical features
Humans. A furuncle may form at the site of the bite. The acute phase lasts about a year, during which the parasites

1

are confined to the blood and lymphatics. There is recurrent fever with severe headache, insomnia, lymphadenititis, anaemia and hyperaesthesia over tibiae. The eyelids and joints may swell and there may also be a rash. In the chronic phase the parasite invades the central nervous system causing progressive mental deterioration, sleepiness during daytime, and neurological signs including convulsions and coma.

Animals. Occasionally mild disease occurs in domestic animals with chronic nervous sequelae in *T. gambiense* infection.

Pathology
Humans. Anaemia and thrombocytopenia are features. Progressive chronic leptomeningitis and glomerulonephritis also occur.

Animals. None.

Special investigations
Humans and animals. Identify trypanosomes by microscopy of lymph-node puncture fluid, capillary blood or buffy coat in the acute phase and of cerebrospinal fluid in the chronic stage. Serological tests include fluorescent antibody, ELISA, indirect haemagglutination and complement fixation tests.

Prognosis
Humans. Untreated illness progresses for 1–2 years until death.

Animals. Usually subclinical.

Prevention
Humans. This involves either reduction of the parasite population by treating humans, avoidance of bites, or vector control by (a) destroying habitat, (b) trapping of tsetse flies and use of insecticides locally, and (c) spraying of insecticides from aircraft. In epidemics, movement of population to safer areas may be warranted.

Animals. Tsetse fly control.

Treatment
Humans. Suramin is used for *T. b. rhodesiense* and pentamidine for *T. b. gambiense* early in the course of illness. Melarsoprol is of possible value for the CNS stage.

Animals. None.

Legislation
Humans. In some endemic areas the disease may be notifiable and movement of untreated patients may be restricted.

Animals. None.

American trypanosomiasis

[Chagas' disease, Chagas–Mazza disease, South American trypanosomiasis]

A common and often fatal protozoal infection of humans in the southern states of the USA and South America. Young children are mainly affected. The disease is usually transmitted by biting insects.

The causative agent is *Trypanosoma cruzi* (Protozoa). There is no vaccine.

Reservoir and mode of transmission
Dogs, cats and guinea pigs are the main reservoirs for human infection. The trypanosome has a complex life-cycle with several transformations in the vertebrate hosts and in the vector. Humans are infected when the insect's faeces become rubbed into the wound caused by the bite of an infected blood-sucking insect (triatomid) or when the conjunctivae, mucous membranes or abrasions become contaminated. After invading local reticulo-endothelial cells the trypanosome multiples in the blood. Adaptation of triatomid vector to the human domestic environment allows transfer of infection between animals, from animals to humans or from human to human. Transmission by blood transfusions from infected persons, congenital

infection, breast milk and laboratory accidents are possible.

Incubation period
Humans. 5–14 days after bite, 30–40 days after blood transfusion.

Animals. 5–42 days.

Clinical features
Humans. Acute illness usually occurs in children with a furuncle at the site of infection. Signs include fever, malaise, enlarged lymph nodes, liver and spleen. If the primary site of infection is the eye there is unilateral oedema of eyelids and conjunctivitis (Romana's sign). Rarely myocarditis and meningoencephalitis occur. Chronic symptoms in adults result from arrhythmias and dilation of the heart, oesophagus and colon.

Animals. Acute and inapparent infection occur in wild animals and chronic disease is seen in dogs. The acute form, which includes fever, enlarged liver and lymph nodes and heart irregularities, lasts 10–30 days before becoming chronic without further clinical signs, though sometimes myocarditis occurs.

Pathology
Humans. Furuncles (chagoma) appear at the point of entry of the infection. Enlarged liver and spleen, myocarditis, grossly dilated heart, intestines, oesophagus, ureter and bladder and meningoencephalitis occur.

Animals. Lesions in dogs resemble those in humans.

Special investigations
Humans and animals. In acute illness identify trypansomes in blood microscopically, or culture by inoculation of blood into suckling mice. Serological tests include fluorescent antibody, ELISA, indirect haemagglutination, complement fixation and latex agglutination tests.

Prognosis
Humans. The fatality rate may approach 8 per cent in infected children.

Animals. In dogs, latent infection may last for years, though myocarditis may shorten the life-span.

Prevention
Humans. Destroy the vector by insecticides or by altering its habitat. Use insect nets to prevent bites. Screen blood donors for infection or treat blood with gentian violet before use. Apply strict laboratory safety precautions.

Animals. Control vectors using insecticides.

Treatment
Humans. Trypanocides may be of use but require expert assessment.

Animals. None.

Legislation
Humans. Notifiable in some endemic areas.

Animals. None.

Ancylostomiasis

[Uncinariasis, necatoriasis, hookworm disease, hookworm anaemia]

A common worm infection of humans and domestic dogs and cats in various tropical and subtropical countries where disposal of human faeces is inadequate. The severity of symptoms depends on the number of worms present.

The causative agents are mainly *Necator americanus* and *Ancylostoma duodenale*; occasionally *A. ceylanicum* and *A. caninum* (Nematoda). There is no vaccine.

Reservoir and mode of transmission
Adult worms, living in the small intestines of humans and animals (dogs and cats), produce eggs which pass on to the ground in faeces. The eggs hatch and go through three

larval stages. Human infection results from the third-stage larvae which survive in soils for several weeks in moist and warm conditions. Animals and man become infected by contact with infected soil, the larvae penetrating through skin or mucosa of the digestive tract. The parasites then migrate through the blood capillaries to the lung, eventually to be coughed up and swallowed. They reach maturity and complete their cycle in the intestines.

Incubation period
Humans and animals.   Variable, up to many months.

Clinical features
Humans.   The condition is often asymptomatic. Self-limiting vesicular/pustular skin eruptions may appear at the site of larval entry. *A. caninum* does not penetrate human skin beyond the epidermis. With other species chronic symptoms due to iron deficiency anaemia may occur. Rarely there is tracheitis and coughing due to lung infiltration with parasites.

Animals.   Factors such as the weight of infection and nutritional state of the animal are important. Loss of blood together with malnutrition produce anaemia. Severe enteritis causes haemorrhagic diarrhoea and weight loss from intestinal malabsorption. Prenatal infection of the dog causes death of the fetal pups. Mild infections generally cause no clinical signs.

Pathology
Humans.   The major disorder is iron deficiency anaemia caused by the leaching of blood. Migration of larvae produces mild skin inflammation at the site of larval entry, and in the lungs. More extensive cutaneous larva migrans is possible. Attachment of the parasites to the wall of the intestine may cause local enteritis and haemorrhage. Eosinophilia is prominent.

Animals.   Anaemia and emaciation occur.

Special investigations
Humans and animals.   Identify hookworms in faeces.

Species differentiation requires examination of adult worms or larvae cultured from faeces.

Prognosis
Humans. Symptoms depend on the weight of infection. Repeated infections are common. Chronic anaemia and developmental retardation are possible.

Animals. Severe anaemia and failure to thrive are likely in the young.

Prevention
Humans. Prevent exposure to larvae by wearing shoes and introduce sanitary methods for disposal of faeces. Screen faeces from persons from endemic areas, and treat cases.

Animals. Keep kennel floors dry, avoid putting out feed for dogs on ground wet with dew when larvae are active.

Treatment
Humans. Mebendazole, pyrantel, bephenium, tetrachloroethylene, iron supplements.

Animals. Oral administration of bephenium compounds.

Legislation
Humans. Not usually notifiable.

Animals. None.

Anisakiasis

[Herring worm disease]

A common parasitic infection from fish. The parasites are widely distributed. Human disease occurs where people eat raw or lightly smoked or salted saltwater fish or squid (e.g. in Japan, the Netherlands, Scandinavia and Central America).

The causative agents are *Anisakis, Phocanema* and *Contracaecum* (Nematoda). There is no vaccine.

Reservoir and mode of transmission
Definitive hosts are marine mammals such as dolphins or seals. These pass the parasite's eggs in their faeces. The eggs hatch and produce larvae which infect the first intermediate host, usually a crustacean. A fish may be the second intermediate host. Humans are aberrant hosts infected by eating fish.

Incubation period
Humans and animals.   A few hours to a few weeks.

Clinical features
Humans.   There may be fever, abdominal pain, vomiting, haematemesis, coughing, pseudoappendicitis, and possibly symptoms associated with intestinal perforation.

Animals.   Fish fail to thrive if heavily infected.

Pathology
Humans.   The larvae usually remain in the intestine causing few lesions. However, they sometimes invade the stomach wall causing haematemesis and may lodge in the mesenteric veins or in the viscera where they induce eosinophilic granulomas and abscesses. Larvae may migrate up the oesophagus to the oropharynx. There is a low-grade eosinophilia.

Animals.   In fish, atrophy of the liver occurs and sometimes fatal infection of the heart. Visceral adhesions and muscle damage can be severe.

Special investigations
Humans.   Identify larvae in the oropharynx or stomach.

Animals.   Demonstrate the parasite in tissues of fish.

Prognosis
Humans.   The condition is rarely fatal.

Animals.   Wide distribution of the parasites and consequent disease results in difficulty in maintaining marine vertebrates in laboratories.

Prevention
Humans. Avoid raw or undercooked fish. Freezing fish kills larvae. Eviscerate fish immediately after catching.

Animals. Impractical.

Treatment
Humans. Physical removal of larvae by gastroscopy or surgery.

Animals. Not appropriate.

Legislation
Humans and animals. None.

Anthrax

[Malignant pustule, wool-sorters' disease, charbon, malignant oedema, splenic fever]

An acute bacterial infection of humans and animals which may be rapidly fatal. The disease occurs worldwide and is enzootic in certain African and Asian countries. It is an occupational hazard of persons such as wool-sorters, fellmongers, knackermen, farm workers and veterinarians in contact with infected animals or their products (e.g. blood, wool, hides and bones).
    The causative agent is *Bacillus anthracis* (bacterium).

Reservoir and mode of transmission
All domestic, zoo and wild animals are potentially at risk of infection. Anthrax bacilli are released from infected carcasses and form resistant spores on exposure to air. These spores contaminate soil for many years. Humans are usually infected by inoculation from direct contact with infected animals, carcasses or animal products and contaminated soil. Inhalation or ingestion of spores may occur. Animals are infected from contaminated feed, forage, water or carcasses. Laboratory accidents have occurred.

Incubation period
Humans.   Cutaneous 3–10 days; inhalation 1–5 days; gastrointestinal 2–5 days.

Animals.   1–5 days.

Clinical features
Humans.   Various forms include:

* Cutaneous anthrax; localized ulceration and scab with fever and headache which may be followed within a few days by septicaemia and meningitis.
* Inhalation anthrax; fulminating pneumonia.
* Intestinal anthrax; acute gastroenteritis with bloody diarrhoea.

Animals.   Peracute cases are found dead or moribund. Acute cases show fever, excitation followed by depression, uncoordination, convulsion and death. Chronic cases show oedema of throat, pharynx and brisket, especially in pigs.

Pathology
Humans.   Features include black scab (eschar) with oedema, enlargement of regional lymph nodes and possibly septicaemia; pneumonia and generalized haemorrhages.

Animals.   Carcasses should not be opened, hence necropsy is rarely carried out. Main features include failure of the blood to clot and haemorrhages throughout the body. The spleen is enlarged and softened. The subcutaneous swelling, mainly about the neck and throat of affected pigs and horses, contains gelatinous fluid. The blood contains very large numbers of *B. anthracis*.

Special investigations
Humans.   Identify *B. anthracis* in stained blood smears or by inoculation of laboratory animals. Culture swabs from wounds.

Animals.   As for humans. Specific antigen for anthrax may be found in animal products (e.g. hides) using a precipitin (Ascoli) test.

Prognosis

Humans. Untreated cutaneous anthrax has a fatality rate of 5–20 per cent and gastrointestinal anthrax of 25–75 per cent. Pulmonary anthrax is usually fatal.

Animals. The condition is usually fatal in cattle unless treated early. Pigs and horses are more resistant.

Prevention

Humans. Prohibit contact with infected animals and their products. Establish environmental and personal hygiene (e.g. ventilation and protective clothing) where a special risk exists. Treat wounds promptly and disinfect imports of hairs and wool. Vaccination may protect those occupationally exposed to risk. Apply strict laboratory safety measures. Isolate infected patients, with concurrent disinfection.

Animals. Sterilize, or avoid using, meat and bone meal from high-risk countries for animal feed. Vaccinate livestock grazing in enzootic area. Dispose of infected carcasses safely and fence off areas contaminated by inadequately buried carcasses.

Treatment

Humans. Antibiotic treatment, especially penicillin.

Animals. Penicillin injection of all animals showing fever after the first case is confirmed. This involves checking temperatures twice daily.

Vaccination

Humans. Offered to workers at risk.

Animals. Non-encapsulated Stern strain vaccine can be used in all species of domestic animal. Annual vaccination of grazing animals using spore or alum precipitated antigen vaccine in areas of high risk is recommended.

Legislation

Humans. The disease is notifiable in most countries. It is a recognized occupational disease in some countries, including the UK.

Animals.   Notifiable in many countries with mandatory disposal of infected carcasses by burning or deep burial under lime. Opening or moving suspect carcasses is prohibited.

Argentine haemorrhagic fever

[Junin disease, Mal de rastrojos, O'Higgins' disease, gripon, north-east Buenos Aires haemorrhagic viraemia, endoepidemic haemorrhagic viraemia]

A viral haemorrhagic fever carried by rodents and affecting mainly farm workers in Argentina, in the wet pampas area used for cereal cultivation.

The causative agent is Junin virus (Arenaviridae). There is no vaccine.

Reservoir and mode of transmission
The reservoir is wild rodents, principally *Calomys musculinus*, which live around cultivated fields. Virus is excreted in the urine and saliva. Transmission is possibly airborne from dust contaminated with rodent excreta, or oral from contaminated food or by direct contact of virus with skin abrasions. Illness in humans coincides with peak rodent populations during the maize harvest from April to July. The virus poses a major hazard to laboratory workers.

Incubation period
Humans.   7–16 days.

Animals.   Unknown.

Clinical features
Humans.   There is an illness of 1–2 weeks with insidious onset of fever, malaise, rigors, fatigue, headache, vomiting, constipation or diarrhoea, conjunctival congestion, retro-orbital pain, epistaxis, petechial haemorrhages beneath skin, palate and gums. Oedema of the upper body is possible. In severe cases haematemesis and melaena, encephalopathy, bradycardia and hypertension occur.

Animals.   Wild rodents show no signs of infection. Guinea pigs experimentally infected develop haemorrhagic fever and die.

Pathology
Humans.   Main changes involve petechiae, leucopaenia, thrombocytopenia, focal liver necrosis and renal tubular necrosis with albuminuria and cellular casts in urine.

Animals.   No known lesion occur in wild rodents. In experimental guinea pigs multiple haemorrhages occur, espccially in the alimentary tract.

Special investigations
Humans.   Isolate virus from the blood or pharyngeal washings in laboratories with maximum containment facilities. Serological tests include indirect fluorescent antibody and complement fixation tests.

Animals.   Post mortem examination not generally carried out.

Prognosis
Humans.   The fatality rate is 5–30 per cent and survivors have prolonged convalesence.

Animals.   Infection in wild rodents is chronic with persistent viraemia.

Prevention
Humans.   Rodent control is the first line of prevention. Take maximum safety precautions in the laboratory. Isolate acutely ill patients and apply concurrent disinfection.

Animals.   None.

Treatment
Humans.   Specific immunoglobulin and symptomatic therapy.

Animals.   None applicable.

Legislation
Humans.   Viral haemorrhagic disease is notifiable in some countries, including the UK.

Animals.   None.

Ascariasis

[Roundworm infection, ascaridiasis]

A common, but usually mild, roundworm infection of both humans and animals, occuring worldwide. There is doubt whether the worms cross between species.

The causative agent in humans is usually *Ascaris lumbricoides*. *Ascaris suum* in pigs is considered occasionally a zoonotic infection (Nematoda). There is no vaccine.

Reservoir and mode of transmission
A. lumbricoides has its reservoir in humans and in contaminated soil. *A. suum* occurs in pigs. Eggs are passed in faeces and become infective after two weeks. Infection is by the ingestion of eggs in soil or undercooked food. Eggs hatch in the gut, penetrate its wall and reach the lungs via the blood stream. Larvae develop in the lungs, ascend the trachea and are swallowed and mature in the gut. Egg-laying begins 45–60 days after initial infection.

Incubation period
Humans.   About two months.

Animals.   Development of *A. suum* in the pig is said to be quicker than in the human.

Clinical features
Humans.   The condition is usually asymptomatic but there may be fever with asthma, spasmodic coughing and possibly pneumonitis. Abdominal pain, and even bowel or bile duct obstruction, is possible. Occasionally migrating larvae cause symptoms referable to the brain, eyes, kidneys and liver.

Animals. Migrating larvae cause irregular breathing and coughing. Heavy infection gives abdominal pain with diarrhoea. Suckling pigs are most affected.

Pathology
Humans. Eosinophilia and pulmonary eosinophilic infiltration occur. Liver abscesses and cholangitis are sometimes seen.

Animals. Larvae migrating through the lung cause pneumonia. Worms in the intestine give enteritis.

Special investigations
Humans. Identify eggs or adult worms in faeces. Larvae in sputum or gastric washings are diagnostic.

Animals. Examine faeces for eggs, or monitor worms passed rectally or via mouth and nose. An egg count of more than 1000/g of faeces indicates clinical disease.

Prognosis
Humans. The condition is rarely fatal. Aberrant larvae in brain, eyes and kidney can give severe symptoms.

Animals. Rarely fatal.

Prevention
Humans. Sanitary disposal of faeces coupled with good personal and food hygiene are essential.

Animals. Worm and wash sows before farrowing. Rear pigs on concrete or avoid close confinement on soil.

Treatment
Humans and animals. Treat periodically with anthelmintics such as levamisole, mebendazole, albendazole, thiobendazole, pyrantel, bephenium and piperazine.

Legislation
Humans and animals. None.

Asian ixodo rickettsiosis

[North Asian tick-borne rickettsiosis, North Asian tick typhus, Siberian tick typhus]

A relatively mild rickettsial fever spread by ticks from wild rodents, in the USSR and Mongolia.

The causative agent is *Rickettsia siberica* (rickettsia). There is no vaccine.

Reservoir and mode of transmission
The reservoir is wild rodents and their ticks. Human infection usually occurs in field workers in the spring during greatest tick activity. Transmission is by tick bite and possibly from inhalation, or contamination of wounds and mucous membranes by tick faeces.

Incubation period
Humans.   2–7 days.

Animals.   Unknown.

Clinical features
Humans.   Illness lasts 1–3 weeks, beginning with sudden onset of fever and chills, severe headache and regional lymphadenitis, which is followed within five days by a pink papular rash.

Animals.   Unknown.

Pathology
Humans.   No specific lesions.

Animals.   Unknown.

Special investigations
Humans.   Isolate the organism by inoculation of laboratory rodents. Serological tests include the Weil–Felix and complement fixation tests.

Animals.   Impracticable.

Prognosis
Humans.   Usually self-limiting and benign.

Animals.   Uncertain.

Prevention
Humans.   Control the tick vector. Avoid tick infested areas and tick bites.

Animals.   Impracticable.

Treatment
Humans.   Symptomatic therapy.

Animals.   Inappropriate.

Legislation
Humans.   Notifiable in some European countries.

Animals.   None.

Babesiosis

[Babesiasis, piroplasmosis, red water fever (in cattle)]

A severe and common protozoal infection of cattle spread occasionally to humans by tick bites.

The causative agents are *Babesia microti* (in north-east USA), *B. bovis* and *B. divergens* (in Europe) and other babesia species (Protozoa).

Reservoir and mode of transmission
The main reservoir is rodents for *B. microti* and cattle for *B. bovis* and *B. divergens*. Infected nymphal ticks bite and transmit infection to humans. Transmission by blood transfusion from human to human is possible.

Incubation period
Humans and animals.   1–12 months.

Clinical features
Humans. Signs include fever, fatigue, haemolytic anaemia, jaundice, haemoglobinuria and renal failure.

Symptoms are more severe and may rapidly progress to death if the patient has had a splenectomy or is immunocompromised.

Animals.   As for the human but many animals show only mild fever and recover spontaneously. Others progress to severe debilitating disease and death.

Pathology
Humans.   Organisms can be seen in red blood cells. Intravascular haemolysis occurs with disseminated intravascular thrombosis.

Animals.   Deaths, which commonly occur in cattle, are due to either anaemic anoxia or pulmonary thrombosis. Other lesions stem from the haemolysis and include enlarged spleen, liver and haemoglobinuric nephrosis.

Special investigations
Humans and animals.   Identify parasites in erythrocytes in blood smears. Isolate by inoculation of blood into susceptible animals: susceptibility may be increased by splenectomy. Serological tests include the indirect fluorescent antibody test.

Prognosis
Humans.   The condition may be fatal in splenectomized or in immunocompromised patients.

Animals.   Acquired immunity is strong. Innate resistance varies amongst races of cattle and increases with age. Fatality rate may reach 90 per cent in susceptible animals introduced into an infected area.

Prevention
Humans.   Control rodents and avoid tick bites.

Animals.   In enzootic areas control, but do not eradicate, the tick population to maintain a low level of infection in indigenous stock, resulting in strong acquired immunity. Vaccinate or treat introduced stock until immunity is established. In redwater-free areas eradicate ticks and prevent introduction of babesia by quarantine of imported livestock.

Treatment
Humans. Clindamycin with quinine has been suggested. Exchange transfusion may be necessary in asplenic patients.

Animals. In cattle, injection of quinuronium compounds, acridine derivatives, aromatic diamines and imidocarb; in sheep, diminazine; in horses, imidocarb.

Vaccination
Humans. None.

Animals. Killed and live attenuated vaccines are available for cattle and sheep.

Legislation
Humans. None.

Animals. Notifiable in cattle in Morocco, Tanzania, Zambia, much of South America, Guatemala, Jamaica, Finland, Lebanon, Israel, Jordan, Oman, Korea, Japan and New Zealand.

Banzi fever

[Germiston fever]

A viral fever probably transmitted by mosquitoes from wild rodents. Only a few human cases have been identified, in southern Africa, although serological surveys suggest more widespread infection.

The causative agents are Banzi virus and Germiston fever virus (Togaviridae). There is no vaccine.

Reservoir and mode of transmission
Wild rodents are the reservoir and the cycle of infection is maintained by *Culex rubinotus* mosquitoes. The mode of human infection is unclear, but presumably infection is mosquito-borne. Accidental infection in laboratory accidents has occurred.

Incubation period
Humans.   Uncertain.

Animals.   Unknown.

Clinical features
Humans.   Fever, headache, myalgia, lassitude and weakness.

Animals.   Not known.

Pathology
Humans.   Uncertain.

Animals.   Unknown.

Special investigations
Humans.   Isolate virus from blood; serology.

Animals.   Inappropriate.

Prognosis
Humans.   Uncertain.

Animals.   Unknown.

Prevention
Humans.   Control the vector tick. Apply safety precautions in the laboratory.

Animals.   Impracticable.

Treatment
Humans.   Symptomatic therapy.

Animals.   None.

Legislation
Humans and animals.   None.

Bolivian haemorrhagic fever

[Black typhus, Machupo virus haemorrhagic fever]

A febrile viral disease resembling Argentinian haemorrhagic fever. It is carried by rodents and affects farm workers in north-eastern Bolivia, mainly in rural areas.

The causative agent is Machupo virus (Arenaviridae).

Reservoir and mode of transmission

Rodents of the species *Callomys callosus* are considered to be the natural hosts attracted into houses by food. Direct transmission occurs amongst rodents and to humans via contamination of food or water by rodent urine and possibly by inhaling contaminated dust. Laboratory and hospital infections have been reported.

Incubation period

Humans. 7–16 days.

Animals. Unknown.

Clinical features

Humans. As Argentinian haemorrhagic fever.

Animals. Unknown but probably subclinical.

Pathology

Humans. As Argentinian haemorrhagic fever. Haemorrhages may occur in the gut wall and the central nervous system.

Animals. Unknown but probably none.

Special investigations

Humans and animals. Isolate virus from blood by inoculation of suckling hamsters. Serological tests include the indirect fluorescent antibody and the complement fixation tests.

Prognosis
Humans.   High fatality rates (5–30 per cent) are associated with outbreaks and there is prolonged convalescence of survivors.

Animals.   Rodents are subclinical carriers but with life-long viraemia and virus excretion in some.

Prevention
Humans.   Control of rodents is the first line of prevention. Apply maximum laboratory safety procedures. Hyperimmune globulin may be of value for infected laboratory workers.

Animals.   Impracticable.

Treatment
Humans.   Symptomatic therapy.

Animals.   Not applicable.

Vaccination
Humans.   None at present.

Animals.   Not applicable.

Legislation
Humans.   Viral haemorrhagic disease is notifiable in some countries, including the UK.

Animals.   None.

Borreliosis

[Relapsing fever, tick-borne relapsing fever, spirochaetal fever, vagabond fever, famine fever]

A widely distributed bacterial infection spread from wild rodents by ticks or lice, with high fatality. Tick-borne relapsing fever occurs in Africa, the Americas, Asia and possibly parts of Europe.

The causative agents are *Borrelia recurrentis* and several other borrelia strains (bacterium). There is no vaccine.

Reservoir and mode of transmission

Epidemic louse-borne infection is not considered zoonotic. Endemic tick-borne relapsing fever is transmitted from the natural wild rodent reservoir by tick bites to humans and dogs. Transovarial transmission in ticks occurs. Blood-borne person-to-person and intrauterine transmission have been reported.

Incubation period

Humans. 1–15 days.

Animals. Unknown.

Clinical features

Humans. Sudden onset of fever lasting for 3–5 days ends with a crisis. Then a febrile period of 2–4 days is followed by one to ten or more recurrences of fever accompanied by severe headaches, nausea, vomiting, diarrhoea, jaundice and sometimes a macular rash with bleeding due to thrombocytopenia. Meningitis and cranial nerve involvement are possible.

Animals. Arthritis and fever predominate in infected dogs. The arthritis recurs and may progress to chronic deformity.

Pathology

Humans. Many lesions occur, including enlarged, soft, infarcted spleen, hepatomegaly, haemorrhages in bone marrow and skin, myocarditis, bronchopneumonia, and meningitis.

Animals. Arthritis, especially of the phalangeal joints, occurs with the possiblity of progression to fibrosis of the joint capsule and ankylosis.

Special investigations

Humans. Identify borrelia in thick blood smears. Otherwise isolate the pathogen by inoculation of blood into susceptible animals if possible.

Animals. Inoculate blood or tissues into rats or mice.

Prognosis
Humans. The fatality rate is up to 40 per cent.

Animals. Although fatality is uncommon, the lesions tend to be progressive.

Prevention
Humans and animals. Control tick vectors and prevent tick bites.

Treatment
Humans and animals. Tetracycline, penicillin.

Legislation
Humans. Louse-borne relapsing fever is notifiable to the World Health organization. Tick-borne infection may be notifiable in some countries (e.g. the UK).

Animals. None.

Botulism

[Limberneck (birds), lamziekte (cattle in S. Africa)]

A severe and often fatal toxaemia of humans and animals worldwide, resulting from eating contaminated and improperly preserved food and feed.

The causative agents are toxins A,B,C,D,E,F and G produced by *Clostridium botulinum* (bacterial toxin).

Reservoir and mode of transmission
C. botulinum survives and multiplies in soil, marine sediment and animal and fish intestines. It multiplies in food under anaerobic conditions, producing toxin. Intoxication follows the ingestion of contaminated food or feed which has been inadequately preserved under anaerobic conditions. In the USA the vehicle of intoxication is usually home-canned vegetables and fruits. In Europe, sausages and smoked or preserved meats and fish, and in Japan, fish are the main vehicles.

Incubation period
Humans and animals. Six hours to several days, but usually 12–36 hours.

Clinical features
Humans. The signs of intoxication include nausea, vomiting and abdominal pain, followed rapidly by neurological symptoms including ptosis, blurred vision, paresis and flaccid paralysis. Respiratory failure may cause death within hours or days. A characteristic feature is descending symmetrical flaccid paralysis.

Animals. Muscle paralysis is especially noticeable, with difficulty in eating leading to progressive paralysis. Foals show a 'shaking' syndrome.

Pathology
Humans and animals. No characteristic primary lesions are found.

Special investigations
Humans. Detect toxin in the serum and faeces. Culture suspected foods and gastric aspirates to reveal the contaminating organism.

Animals. As for humans. Test filtrates of stomach and intestinal contents for toxin.

Prognosis
Humans. The fatality rate depends on the dose of toxin ingested and may be high (15–30 per cent), with slow convalescence for survivors.

Animals. As in humans, though the fatality tends to be higher.

Prevention
Humans. Thoroughly treat or reject suspect canned or preserved foods. Refrigerate stored foods. Carefully inspect bottling and canning plants. Health education is needed to promote good food hygiene practices. Urgently investigate cases to identify and remove contaminated foods. Persons

who have eaten implicated food need gastric lavage.

Animals.   Avoid contaminated feed and provide adequate diet to avoid 'pica'. Ensure adequate acid formation during silage making. Vaccinate in enzootic areas.

Treatment
Humans.   Polyvalent antitoxin given early (within 1–2 days of ingestion) may improve prognosis, but risk of severe hypersensitivity reaction to horse serum is high. Give intensive respiratory support.

Animals.   Not usually appropriate. Recovery is possible with careful nursing.

Vaccination
Humans.   None.

Animals.   Toxoid is available.

Legislation
Humans.   The condition is notifiable either specifically or as food poisoning in most countries.

Animals.   None.

Boutonneuse fever

[Marseilles fever, South African tick typhus, Kenya tick typhus, India tick typhus, Mediterranean tick fever]

A mild, tick-borne rickettsial infection of South-East Asia, Africa, India, and countries adjacent to the Mediterranean, Black and Caspian Seas.

The causative agent is *Rickettsia conorii* (rickettsia). There is no vaccine.

Reservoir and mode of transmission
The reservoir is the brown dog tick *Rhipicephalus sanguineus* in the Mediterranean area and a variety of other ticks in other areas. the organism is maintained independently in the tick. There may also be a cycle amongst small wild mammals and their ticks. Humans are accidental hosts

especially at risk from infected dog ticks. Laboratory infections may occur.

Incubation period
Humans. 5–7 days.

Animals. Unknown.

Clinical features
Humans. A primary ulcer with black centre and red edge may occur at the site of the tick bite, followed by swelling of regional lymph nodes and fever, joint and muscle pains and headache, lasting for 1–2 weeks. The conjuctivae may be the site of primary infection with severe conjunctivitis. A maculopapular erythematous rash usually develops within five days over the whole body, including the palms of the hands and sole of the feet; the rash may bleed.

Animals. Unknown, but apparently benign or subclinical in dogs.

Pathology
Humans. Skin ulcers occur with reactive hyperplasia of regional lymph nodes.

Animals. Unknown.

Special investigations
Humans. None is carried out regularly. Serological tests include the Weil–Felix and complement fixation tests.

Animals. As for humans.

Prognosis
Humans. Usually a mild self-limiting infection. The fatality rate is less than 3 per cent.

Animals. Unknown.

Prevention
Humans. Remove ticks from humans and dogs and use tickicides on dogs and their kennels and bedding. Avoid

tick-infested areas. Apply laboratory safety procedures.

Animals.   Impracticable.

Treatment
Humans.   Tetracycline and chloramphenicol.

Animals.   None.

Legislation
Humans.   Notifiable in some European countries.

Animals.   None.

Brucellosis

[In humans: Mediterranean fever, undulant fever, Malta fever. In animals: contagious abortion, epizootic abortion, Bang's disease]

A bacterial infection which may cause recurrent or chronic fever in humans. It is acquired by contact with infected animals or dairy produce. In ruminants and pigs the infection causes abortion.

The causative agents are *Brucella abortus, B. canis, B. melitensis, B. ovis, B. neotomae, B. suis* (bacterium).

B. abortus occurs worldwide but eradication proceeds in developed countries. *B. canis* is widespread in North America. *B. ovis* occurs in New Zealand, Australia, Africa, Europe, North and Central America. *B. melitensis* is enzootic in Mediterranean countries, south-east Russia, Mongolia, the Middle East and Latin America. *B. suis* is enzootic in Latin America and sporadic in Europe, Asia, Africa and Oceania.

Reservoir and mode of transmission
B. abortus in cattle, *B. canis* in dogs, *B. melitensis* in goats, *B. neotomae* in desert rats, *B. ovis* in sheep, *B. suis* in pigs and horses. Transmission amongst animals occurs via contact with infected fetuses, their membranes and fluids which are heavily infected. Subsequent parturitions are heavily infected also. Human infection follows the ingestion of contaminated unpasteurized dairy produce or

following direct contact with infected material (e.g. blood, urine, vaginal discharge) and is an occupational hazard for farm workers and veterinarians. Inhalation of infected material in enclosed spaces is a risk. Person-to-person transmission is rare. Laboratory accidents occur.

Incubation period
Humans. 1–6 weeks, but variable.

Animals. Variable.

Clinical features
Humans. Undulating fever, malaise, weakness, fatigue, rigors, night sweats, headache, backache, joint pains, weight loss and other systemic symptoms occur. Enlarged lymph nodes, liver and spleen, osteomyelitis and endocarditis are possible. Symptoms, including depression, may be wrongly attributed to neuroses, and may persist for months or years with frequent recurrences.

Animals. *B. abortus* in cows causes abortion, often with a retained placenta and ensuing metritis. In bulls, epididymo-orchitis occurs occasionally. Other changes include hygromatous swellings of the knees and arthritis. The disease occurs in outbreaks of 'abortion storms' in which all susceptible cows in a herd abort. In horses the infection localizes in the supraspinous bursae of the neck, leading to chronic suppuration (fistulous withers). In sheep and goats abortion occurs less frequently than in cattle, the main problem being epididymitis in the rams. In pigs, abortion and orchitis occur, together with osteomyelitis of the verte-brae and posterior paralysis.

Pathology
Humans. The condition is characterized by granulomata in lymph nodes, liver, spleen, bone marrow and other sites.

Animals. Brucella localizes intracellularly in the reticulo-endothelial system and provokes a generalized granulomatous reaction. Lymph nodes, spleen and liver enlarge. Joints undergo arthritis with eventual ankylosis. Lesions in the testis and epididymis are of chronic inflammation with degeneration of the seminiferous tubules. In cattle the organisms localize in and destroy the chorioendothelial layer of the placenta.

Special investigations
Humans.   Isolate and type the brucellae from blood or bone marrow. Serological tests include the agglutination test.

Animals.   Isolate brucella from placental material, vaginal swabs and milk by culture or by guinea pig inoculation; serology; milk ring test for agglutinins in cows' milk.

Prognosis
Humans.   Infection may persist, with bouts of undulant fever, for many years. Antibiotics can effect a cure within one year in about 80 per cent of cases. Case fatality if untreated is less than 2 per cent.

Animals.   Abortion is followed by immunity, though carrier state persists especially with secretions from the udder. Fertility is reduced in males with epididymitis.

Prevention
Humans.   Control or preferably eradicate infection from animal reservoirs. Heat-treat all milk. Good personal hygiene is essential and laboratory safety is especially important.

Animals.   Vaccination reduces the prevalence of disease, followed by eradication by test and slaughter. Safely dispose of aborted fetuses and fetal membranes. Test breeding stock in quarantine before importation.

Treatment
Humans.   Antibiotics: especially tetracyclines, streptomycin, trimethoprim and sulphamethoxazole.

Animals.   Not usually attempted.

Vaccination
Humans.   Not very effective and rarely used.

Animals. Live attenuated Strain 19 and killed 45/20 vaccines are commonly used to control *B. abortus* in cattle. Live and killed *B. melitensis* vaccine are available for sheep and goats, and Strain 19 vaccine is claimed to protect against *B. melitensis*.

Legislation
Humans. Notifiable in most countries, including Australia, Canada, New Zealand, the UK and the USA.

Animals. There are official control schemes, often with a slaughter policy, in many countries, including Great Britain, especially for infection in cattle.

Bunyamwera fever

[A mild febrile viral disease of uncertain origin, in Africa south of the Sahara.]

The causative agent is Bunyamwera virus (Bunyaviridae). There is no vaccine.

Reservoir and mode of transmission
The virus has been isolated from mosquitoes and humans but there is only serological evidence of animal infection. Presumably transmission is by mosquito bite.

Incubation period
Humans. Uncertain.

Animals. Unknown.

Clinical features
Humans. Fever, headache and systemic symptoms for up to one week duration.

Animals. Unknown.

Pathology
Humans. There are no characteristic lesions.

Animals. Unknown.

Special investigations
Humans.   Isolate virus from blood; serology.

Animals.   Impracticable.

Prognosis
Humans.   It is apparently a self-limiting acute illness.

Animals.   Unknown.

Prevention
Humans.   Prevent mosquito bites.

Animals.   Impracticable.

Treatment
Humans.   Symptomatic therapy.

Animals.   None.

Legislation
Humans and animals.   None.

Bussuquara fever

Only one human case has been reported, in South America. The causative agent was Bussuquara virus (Togaviridae).

Reservoir and mode of transmission
The natural hosts are wild rodents and mosquitoes and transmission to humans is presumed to arise from mosquito bites.

Incubation period
Humans.   Uncertain.

Animals.   Unknown.

Clinical features
Humans.   Fever and probably systemic symptoms for a few days.

Animals. Unknown.

Pathology
Humans. Uncertain.

Animals. Unknown.

Special investigations
Humans. Isolate virus from blood. Serological tests include the complement fixation, haemagglutination inhibition and neutralization tests.

Animals. None.

Prognosis
Humans. Uncertain.

Animals. Unknown.

Prevention
Humans. Avoid mosquito bites.

Animals. None.

Treatment
Humans. Symptomatic therapy.

Animals. None.

Vaccination
Humans. None.

Animals. Not practicable.

Legislation
Humans and animals. None.

Bwamba fever

A mild febrile viral disease of uncertain origin, in Central and Southern Africa.

The causative agent is Bwamba virus (Bunyaviridae). There is no vaccine.

Reservoir and mode of transmission
Virus has been isolated from humans but there is only serological evidence for infection in mammals and birds. The mode of transmission is uncertain.

Incubation period
Humans.   Uncertain.

Animals.   Unknown.

Clinical features
Humans.   Fever, weakness, and skin rash lasts a few days.

Animals.   Unknown.

Pathology
Humans.   None characteristic.

Animals.   Unknown.

Special investigations
Humans.   Isolate virus from blood. Serological tests include haemagglutination inhibition, complement fixation and neutralization tests.

Animals.   Serology.

Prognosis
Humans.   Usually only a mild or subclinical infection.

Animals.   Unknown.

Prevention
Humans.   None.

Animals.   Impracticable.

Treatment
Humans.   Symptomatic therapy.

Animals.   None.

Legislation
Humans and animals. None.

California encephalitis/La Crosse encephalitis (USA)

[Tahyna virus (Europe)]

A mild, febrile, viral disease which occasionally causes severe encephalitis. It is transmitted by mosquitoes from small wild mammals, mainly in summer, to persons frequenting woodland areas of the USA and Canada, and certain European countries such as Yugoslavia and the USSR.

The causative agents are the California encephalitis group of viruses (Bunyaviridae). There is no vaccine.

Reservoir and mode of transmission
The virus cycles amongst small wild animals (e.g. chipmunks, squirrels, rabbits and hares) and a variety of mosquito species. The infection can be maintained independently over several years by transovarial transmission in the mosquito. Humans are accidental hosts infected by mosquito bite during occupational or recreational activities in wooded areas. Accidental infections from laboratory accidents have occured.

Incubation period
Humans. 5–15 days.

Animals. Unknown.

Clinical features
Humans. Symptoms lasting about 5–10 days range from fever and headache with nausea and vomiting to fits and signs of aseptic meningitis, encephalitis and neurological sequelae.

Animals. Unknown but assumed subclinical.

Pathology
Humans.   Encephalitis.

Animals.   Unknown.

Special investigations
Humans.   Serological tests include the haemagglutination inhibition and neutralization tests.

Animals.   Impracticable.

Prognosis
Humans.   In humans fatality is rare but neurological defects may persist.

Animals.   Thought to be subclinical.

Prevention
Humans.   Prevent mosquito bites. Control the mosquito vector. Apply laboratory safety procedures.

Animals.   Impracticable.

Treatment
Humans.   Symptomatic therapy.

Animals.   Not applicable.

Legislation
Humans.   Acute encephalitis is notifiable in many countries, including the USA and the UK.

Animals.   None.

Campylobacteriosis

[Campylobacter enteritis, vibriosis, vibrionic abortion]

In humans worldwide, a common, enteric, bacterial infection usually transmitted from raw or inadequately cooked food. In animals some strains cause abortion.

The causative agents are *Campylobacter jejuni, C. fetus* and *C. coli* (bacterium).

Reservoir and mode of transmission

There is widespread intestinal carriage in most mammals and birds. The commonest infection in humans is *C. jejuni*. Poultry and cattle are the main reservoirs for human infection, which is acquired by ingesting contaminated raw milk, undercooked chicken or other food contaminated in the kitchen. Direct faecal–oral spread from animals occurs, especially from puppies, and from person to person. Large water-borne outbreaks have occurred.

Incubation period

Humans.   1–10 days, but usually 3–5 days.

Animals.   Unknown because the infection rarely causes enteric disease.

Clinical features

Humans.   There is acute onset of fever, abdominal pain and diarrhoea which may be blood-stained but which usually resolves within ten days. It may cause pseudo-appendicitis and, rarely, septicaemia and arthritis.

Animals.   In cattle and sheep affected by *C. fetus* the main clinical sign is infertility with abortion of the early fetus. *C. jejuni* and *C. coli* may occasionally be associated with diarrhoea in animals, especially when acting secondarily to virus infection.

Pathology

Humans.   Inflammation and ulceration of mucosa of small intestine.

Animals.   Placental necrosis occurs in pregnant cattle.

Special investigations

Humans.   Isolate and type the organism from faeces using

selective media in a CO_2 enriched atmosphere at a temperature of 43°C. Serology may be useful in outbreaks.

Animals. Culture faeces, foods of animal origin and drinking water.

Prognosis
Humans. Usually self-limiting gastroenteritis.

Animals. *C. jejuni* and *C. coli* rarely cause illness in animals. Sometimes isolated from puppies with diarrhoea but significance unknown.

Prevention
Humans. Pasteurize milk. Chlorinate drinking water supplies. Thoroughly cook meat (especially poultry) and practice good kitchen hygiene.

Animals. Prevent introduction of *C. fetus* by restricting purchases to known non-infected virgin animals and use of artificial insemination in cattle.

Treatment
Humans. Give fluid replacement if dehydrated. Erythromycin may help shorten severe infections.

Animals. Treatment is usually unnecessary; it is of doubtful value in *C. jejuni* and *C. coli* carriers. Local and parenteral antibiotic treatment may control venereal infections in bulls and reduce abortions in a newly infected sheep flock.

Vaccination
Humans. None.

Animals. Vaccination may reduce the incidence of infertility in *C. fetus* infections.

Legislation
Humans. The condition is notifiable if thought to be food-poisoning in many countries. Campylobacteriosis

may be notifiable in some countries, including Australia, Israel and New Zealand.

Animals.   *C. fetus* infection is notifiable in some Central and South American and European countries. Slaughter policy operates in Cuba and USSR for *C. fetus*.

Capillariasis

[Capillariosis, intestinal capillariasis, hepatic capillariasis, pulmonary capillariasis]

A roundworm intestinal infection acquired by eating raw fish and which may cause fatal liver disease.

The causative agents are *Capillaria hepatica* (hepatic form), *C. philippinensis* (intestinal form) and *C. aerophila* (respiratory form) (Nematoda). There is no vaccine.

C. hepatica and *C. aerophila* are very rare infections with isolated cases reported from North, Central and South America, Asia and Europe. *C. philippinensis* is endemic in certain areas of the Philippines and cases have been reported from Thailand and Japan.

Reservoir and mode of transmission

Humans are probably the principal reservoir for *C. philippinensis* and are infected by eating raw fish (the intermediate host) containing infective larvae. The worm parasite lives in the intestines of humans and autoinfection occurs. Human faeces contain large numbers of ova which contaminate water-courses and infect freshwater fish. With *C hepatica* rodents are the reservoirs. Cats and dogs are the reservoir of *C. aerophila*. Humans may be infected by the ingestion of ova in the soil.

Incubation period

Humans.   Probably 3–4 weeks.

Animals.   Unknown, but *C. hepatica* ova need two months to embryonate and then one month to mature in a rodent's liver. For *C. philippinensis* the cycle has only recently been clarified, but the incubation period is not yet known.

Clinical features
Humans.   *C. hepatica*: acute and subacute hepatitis. *C. philippinensis*: progressive weight and protein loss due to diarrhoea and malabsorption. *C. aerophila*: fever and coughing.

Animals.   Unknown.

Pathology
Humans.   *C. philippinensis*: the lesions are confined to the small intestine. The jejunal villi are obliterated with massive accumulations of worms and ova. *C. hepatica*: the liver lesions consist of enlargement with foci of granulation tissue containing worms and ova. *C. aerophila*: worms present in epithelial lining of respiratory tract causing pneumonitis.

Animals.   Unknown.

Special investigations
Humans.   *C. hepatica*: Hepatic biopsies reveal nodules containing parasites and eggs. Eggs are not present in faeces. *C. philippinensis*: examine faecal samples for eggs, larvae or adult worms. *C. aerophila*: eggs may appear in sputum or in biopsy specimens.

Animals.   Demonstrate the parasites in rodents or fish at post mortem examination.

Prognosis
Humans.   Fatality rates of up to 10 per cent for untreated *C. philippinensis* occur and the relapse rate is high.

Animals.   Signs of infection in animals are not recognized.

Prevention
Humans.   Control rodents and improve hygiene. Prevent

children eating soil. Sanitary disposal of faeces. Cook fish thoroughly.

Animals. Impractical.

Treatment
Animals. Mebendazole.

Animals. Inappropriate.

Legislation
Humans. May be notifiable in endemic areas.

Animals. None.

Cat scratch disease

[Cat scratch fever, benign lymphoreticulosis]

A prolonged regional lymphadenopathy resulting from cat scratches, presumed to be infective in origin. It occurs worldwide.

The causative agent is unknown, but is possibly a Gram-negative bacillus. There is no vaccine.

Reservoir and mode of transmission
Cats may be the reservoir or merely mechanical carriers. The majority of cases have been bitten or scratched by cats, although some instances followed trauma by inanimate objects.

Incubation period
Humans. 3–14 days.

Animals. Unknown.

Clinical features
Humans. A prolonged or recurrent lymphadenopathy which may last up to two years but which usually resolves within four months. Initially a red papule develops at the site of inoculation. When the site is the eyelid or

conjunctivae, conjunctivitis and periauricular lymphadenitis (Parinaud's oculoglandular syndrome) may follow. Fever, malaise, rash, muscle and joint pains, weight loss and splenomegaly are unusual manifestations.

Animals.   Unknown and probably subclinical.

Pathology
Humans.   Granulomata, which may contain small pleomorphic bacilli demonstrated by Warthin–Starry stain, occur in primary lesions, regional lymph nodes and the spleen. Lymph nodes show reticular-cell hyperplasia and hypertrophy. Necrosis and suppuration of lymph nodes is common.

Animals.   Unknown.

Special investigations
Humans.   Examine histopathology of lymph node biopsies.

Animals.   None.

Prognosis
Humans.   It is usually a self-limiting disease, but recurrent or chronic illness is possible.

Animals.   In all cases the implicated cats have appeared healthy.

Prevention
Humans.   Wash cat scratches immediately.

Animals.   None.

Treatment
Humans.   Symptomatic therapy.

Animals.   None.

Legislation
Humans and animals.   None.

Chikungunya fever

[Chik fever]

A benign, febrile, viral disease transmitted by mosquitoes from wild primates. It can give rise to persistent arthritis. Outbreaks affect rural populations in wooded areas especially in tropical Africa, but also in subtropical Africa, the Philippines, South East Asia and India.

The causative agent is Chik virus (Togaviridae). There is no vaccine.

Reservoir and mode of transmission
The reservoir is probably in wild primates and bats. Transmission is by mosquito vectors which frequent the forest canopy.

Incubation period
Humans. 1–12 days.

Animals. Unknown.

Clinical features
Humans. The disease begins with a sudden onset of fever which lasts for up to two weeks with headache, coryza, severe joint pains, arthritis, conjuctivitis and lymphadenopathy. Fever may be biphasic. A maculopapular rash occurs within 2–5 days of onset. Occasionally haemorrhagic manifestations occur.

Animals. Unknown.

Pathology
Humans. Periarticular nodules of chronic inflammatory reaction.

Animals. Unknown.

Special investigations
Humans. Isolate virus from the blood. Serological tests include the haemagglutination inhibition, complement fixation and neutralization tests.

Animals.   Impracticable.

Prognosis
Humans. Though usually self-limiting, convalescence may be prolonged with persistent arthritis and severe pains in the joints.

Animals.   Unknown, but probably subclinical.

Prevention
Humans.   Control mosquitoes and avoid their bites.

Animals.   Inappropriate.

Treatment
Humans.   Symptomatic therapy.

Animals.   Impracticable.

Legislation
Humans and animals.   None.

Chlamydiosis

[Psittacosis, ornithosis, parrot fever]

A febrile bacterial disease acquired by contact with infected birds and rarely animals. It occurs worldwide.

The causative agent is *Chlamydia psittaci* (obligatory intracellular bacterium).

Reservoir and mode of transmission
Psittacine and other birds, including ducks, turkeys and pigeons, are the usually identified source of human infections. Ovine strains may infect pregnant women. Infection is via inhalation of aerosols or of infected dust contaminated by bird faeces, nasal discharges, or sheep products of gestation or abortion. *C. psittaci* may survive in dust for many months. Person-to-person transmission of avian or ovine strains is rare. Outbreaks occur amongst aviary and quarantine station workers, poultry processing workers and veterinarians.

Incubation period
Humans.   Usually 4–15 days.

Animals.   Unknown.

Clinical features
Humans.   The disease varies from an influenza-like illness with fever, headache, joint and muscle pains of a few days duration to atypical pneumonia and possibly endocarditis and hepatitis lasting several weeks.

Animals.   Often asymptomatic, but fever, diarrhoea, anorexia, respiratory distress, conjunctivitis and nasal discharge are possible.

Pathology
Humans.   Patchy infiltration of the lungs occurs, possibly leading to bronchopneumonia. Vegetations may develop on damaged heart valves.

Animals.   Oedema of the lungs occurs and the pleural and peritoneal cavities fill with fibrinous exudate. Liver and spleen enlarge.

Special investigations
Humans.   Serological tests used are the complement fixation and indirect fluorescent antibody tests. Isolation of *C. psittaci* is not usually attempted.

Animals.   Demonstrate the organism in stained smears of liver and spleen from birds, or placentae from sheep. Isolation in tissue culture can be attempted from post mortem tissues and avian faeces.

Prognosis
Humans.   Fatality from avian chlamydiosis in humans is rare. Ovine chlamydial infection in pregnant women is life-threatening, causing late abortion or neonatal death and disseminated intravascular coagulation in the mother.

Animals.   Most infections are inapparent except for abortion in sheep and respiratory disease in parrots.

Prevention
Humans.   Quarantine infected birds. Provide good ventilation of poultry processing plants. Heat-treat feathers. Educate exposed workers. Safely dispose of infected birds. Pregnant women should avoid contact with flocks during lambing in enzootic areas. Apply strict laboratory safety procedures when handling avian strains.

Animals.   Prevention is difficult in poultry because of reintroduction of infection by wild birds. Give prolonged tetracycline treatment to imported birds in quarantine in the feed to eliminate carriage. In sheep, keep flocks closed or vaccinate annually. Isolate aborting ewes until discharges cease.

Treatment
Humans.   Tetracycline and erythromycin.

Animals.   Give oxytetracycline in the feed of pet birds. Prolonged treatment is needed to eliminate carriage.

Vaccination
Humans.   None.

Animals.   Live attenuated vaccine is available for sheep.

Legislation
Humans.   The disease may be notifiable in some countries, including Australia, New Zealand, the USA and several European countries, but excluding the UK.

Animals.   There is control of the importation of birds, and compulsory quarantine and treatment. The disease is notifiable in poultry in some countries of Africa, Central and South America, Europe including the UK, and the Middle East. Chlamydial abortion in sheep is notifiable in a few countries.

Clonorchiasis

[Chinese liver fluke disease]

A usually asymptomatic parasitic disease of the liver of humans, dogs and cats, caused by eating raw fish. It occurs in China, especially the south-east, South Korea, Japan, Taiwan and Vietnam.

The causative agent is *Clonorchis sinensis* (Trematoda). There is no vaccine.

Reservoir and mode of transmission
The complete life-cycle includes two intermediate hosts, a gastropod snail and several species of freshwater fish. Humans or other definitive hosts (mainly cats and dogs) pass embryonated eggs in the faeces. These hatch in the snail's intestine and pass through larval stages, multiply and eventually form cercaria which swim free and penetrate freshwater fish in which they encyst. Humans and other definitive hosts are infected when they eat raw fish. The adults live and complete their life-cycle in the bile ducts.

Incubation period
Humans and animals.   Variable.

Clinical features
Humans.   The condition is often asymptomatic, but symptoms due to obstruction of bile ducts may occur. They include anorexia, abdominal discomfort, hepatomegaly, jaundice and cirrhosis.

Animals.   Fever, enlarged liver and jaundice in dogs and cats.

Pathology
Humans.   There is obstruction of bile ducts leading to

cholangitis, portal cirrhosis, and possibly to carcinoma of the liver; eosinophilia.

Animals.   As for humans. The disease may initiate biliary lithiasis.

Special investigations
Humans and animals.   Identify eggs in faeces.

Prognosis
Humans.   Depending on the weight of infection the outcome may be asymptomatic or lead to cirrhosis and death.

Animals.   Light infections are asymptomatic.

Prevention
Humans.   Cook, freeze or salt freshwater fish. Sanitary disposal of faeces.

Animals.   Cook or freeze fish thoroughly before feeding to cats and dogs.

Treatment
Humans.   Praziquantel.

Animals.   Chloroquine or praziquantel.

Legislation
Humans and animals.   None.

Clostridial diseases

[Clostridial myositis: black leg, malignant oedema, gas gangrene. Enterotoxaemia: pulpy kidney, struck, lamb dysentery, braxy. Tetanus (lockjaw)]

A group of diseases occuring worldwide, caused by toxins produced by anaerobic, sporeforming clostridial bacteria. Disease is manifest by signs of necrotizing myositis, enterotoxaemia or paralysis, depending on the causal organism.

The causative agents are *Clostridium perfringens,*

Cl. chauvoei, Cl. novyi, Cl. septicum, Cl. tetani and other clostridial species (bacterium).

Reservoir and mode of transmission
Clostridia are normal intestinal flora and also survive by spores in the soil. Infection may be by contamination of deep, penetrating wounds to cause tetanus, by ingestion of preformed toxin or spores which vegetate in the digestive tract to cause enterotoxaemia, or by ingestion of spores which are carried by the blood to muscles where they remain dormant until activated by trauma to produce necrotizing myositis. *Cl. perfringens* food poisoning is due to spore contamination of foods which survive heating to vegetate in unrefrigerated conditions. Neonatal tetanus in humans is frequently caused by contamination of the umbilicus.

Incubation period
Humans. Gas gangrene: a few hours to several days. Tetanus: variable, usually 3–21 days. Food poisoning: 6–24 hours.

Animals. Variable.

Clinical features
Humans. Tetanus: painful toxic contractions of muscles and trismus. Gas gangrene: fever, toxaemia, painful oedema spreading from the edges of wounds, interstitial emphysema, neck stiffness. Food poisoning: vomiting and diarrhoea of a few days' duration.

Animals. Tetanus: as in humans. In myositis (black leg) cases a limb is stiff and painful with crepitus on palpation. Signs of toxaemia. Rapidly fatal.

Pathology
Humans. Gas gangrene: darkening of infected tissue, gas formation in tissue and spreading necrosis due to the effect of toxin.

Animals. *Cl. chauvoei, Cl. novyi* and *Cl. septicum* toxins produce massive muscle necrosis, often with oedema and subcutaneous gas formation. *Cl. perfringens* causes a variety of profound toxaemias with cloudy swelling of parenchymatous organs and excess fluid, often blood-stained or containing a plasma clot, in serous cavities. In pulpy kidney disease of lambs the renal cortex can be washed away under running water.

Special investigations
Humans.   Culture of the organism from patients is rarely helpful unless related to food isolates in suspected food-poisoning.

Animals.   Stain smears of affected muscle exudate to show Gram-positive bacilli in profusion. Spore position and size within the bacillus may indicate the species. Fluorescent antibody stains are available to identify. *Cl. novyi, Cl. septicum* and *Cl. chauvoei.* Toxin in gut contents may be demonstrated by intravenous inoculation of extracts into mice.

Prognosis
Humans.   Gas gangrene has a high fatality if untreated. The case fatality rate for tetanus is 30–90 per cent even when treated. Food-poisoning is usually self-limiting.

Animals.   Clostridial toxaemia is usually fatal in unvaccinated animals.

Prevention
Humans.   Clean wounds thoroughly and always sterilize surgical instruments. Routinely immunize children and give antitoxin after wounding if the patient was not immunized. Booster doses of tetanus toxoid are necessary if ten years have elapsed since the last dose. Good food hygiene is essential.

Animals.   Prevent wound contamination during lambing, shearing, castration and docking. On farms where clostridial disease recurs, cattle between six months and two years of age should be vaccinated at least two months before the period of risk, usually in spring and summer. Breeding sheep should be vaccinated annually in late pregnancy, and lambs which are to be kept for breeding should be vaccinated at three months of age.

Treatment

Humans.   Radical surgery of infected wounds is needed, and antibiotic therapy (e.g. penicillin with use of antitoxin). Provision of hyperbaric oxygen may help.

Animals.   Large doses of intravenous crystalline penicillin followed by longer acting preparations may save a proportion of tetanus or blackleg cases if given early.

Vaccination

Humans.   Routine tetanus toxoid immunization is best given in childhood. Booster doses in adults are needed especially following injury. Passive immunization with specific immunoglobulin is used in unimmunized.

Animals.   Killed vaccines are usually given in combination against all the prevalent clostridial diseases of the area.

Legislation

Humans.   Tetanus and food-poisoning are notifiable in most countries.

Animals.   Blackleg is notifiable in some countries of Africa, Central and South America, Asia and Europe including the Channel Isles, but not Great Britain. Slaughter policy for cattle in the Channel Isles, Belgium, Romania and for sheep and cattle in Luxembourg, Korea and Japan.

Coenurosis

[Coenuriasis, gid (in sheep)]

A rare parasitic disease in humans which may cause severe and slowly progressive disease caused by the intermediate stage of a dog tapeworm.

The causative agents are *Coenurus cerebralis, C. serialis* and *C. brauni* (Cestoda). There is no vaccine.

C. cerebralis and *C. serialis* occur worldwide in temperate climates. *C. brauni* occurs only in Africa.

Reservoir and mode of transmission

Definitive hosts are dogs and wild canidae. Intermediate hosts of *C. cerebralis* are sheep in which the larval form occurs in the brain. *C. serialis* occurs in the connective tissues of rabbits and hares and *C. brauni* in wild rodents. Gravid proglottids with eggs are excreted from the definitive hosts and the intermediate host is infected by ingesting these eggs from the contaminated environment. The parasite penetrates and grows into a large cyst. The cycle completes when dogs consume infected tissue of the intermediate host containing the cysts.

Incubation period

Humans. Uncertain but sometimes prolonged.

Animals. Varies depending on the growth rate of the parasite and its location in sheep. In dogs no clinical signs occur.

Clinical features

Humans. There may be the neurological consequences of brain cysts (e.g. paraplegia). Cysts in the eye give pain and loss of vision.

Animals. Clinical signs vary depending on the location of the coenuri in the brain of sheep. They include circular movements, uncoordination, paralysis and convulsions. Mortality is high.

Pathology

Humans. There is meningoencephalitis owing to the invasion of the parasite cysts and their pressure effects on the brain. In humans, aberrant forms of the cysts develop in the eye (ophthalmic coenurus) with chorioretinal lesions.

Animals. Encephalitis from the trauma of the migrating parasite.

Special investigations

Humans. Biopsy affected tissue to identify the parasite.

Animals. Examine dog faeces for tapeworms and their eggs after purging.

Prognosis
Humans. Poor with little hope for complete recovery.

Animals. The tapeworm has little effect on dogs but mortality in sheep showing nervous signs is high.

Prevention
Humans. Adopt strict personal hygiene. Prevent dogs fouling the environment and vegetables, etc. Worm all dogs.

Animals. Prevent dogs from eating carcasses of intermediate hosts, and cook offal before feeding.

Treatment
Humans. Probably albendazole and praziquantel may be useful.

Animals. Tapeworms can be eliminated from dogs by oral arecoline hydrobromide or praziquantel. Removing cysts from the brain of affected sheep by trephining has been attempted but is rarely worthwhile.

Legislation
Humans and animals. None.

Colorado tick fever

[Mountain fever]

A febrile viral disease transmitted by ticks from small rodents, in the north-western states of the USA, British Columbia and Alberta. Though usually benign it can cause encephalitis in children.

The causative agent is Colorado tick fever virus (Reoviridae). There is no vaccine.

Reservoir and mode of transmission
These include small wild animals and ticks. The virus cycles between squirrels and small rodents and the tick, *Dermacentor andersoni*. Virus is transmitted from stage to stage in ticks but not transovarially. Humans are accidental

hosts infected by tick bites during spring and early summer when the ticks are active.

Incubation period
Humans.   3–6 days.

Animals.   Usually subclinical and hence not known.

Clinical features
Humans.   Illness begins with fever of sudden onset with headache, photophobia, muscle and joint pains. This stage lasts about two days and is followed by a remission of 2–3 days and then a second episode of fever for three or more days with a maculopapular rash. Illness is generally benign in adults but can be more severe in children with signs of encephalitis.

Animals.   Subclinical, although viraemia occurs in squirrels.

Pathology
Humans.   Neutropenia and thrombocytopenia are usual and encephalitis and myocarditis may occur with focal necrosis in tissues.

Animals.   Unknown.

Special investigations
Humans.   Isolate virus from the blood. Direct immunofluorescence tests reveal antigen in red blood cells. Serological tests include complement fixation, neutralization and indirect fluorescent antibody tests.

Animals.   Isolate virus in tissue culture or by inoculation of suckling mice; serology.

Prognosis
Humans.   Death is rare, though convalescence can be prolonged.

Animals.   Viraemia in mammals is subclinical.

Prevention
Humans.   Avoid tick infested areas and tick bites by use of protective clothing or repellents. Ensure strict laboratory safety.

Animals.   Control the tick vector.

Treatment
Humans.   Symptomatic therapy.

Animals.   Inappropriate.

Legislation
Humans.   The condition is notifiable in USA and other countries if acute encephalitis.

Animals.   None.

Corynebacterial diseases

A mixed group of comparatively rare infectious disorders of humans, including pharyngitis, wound contamination and pneumonia acquired by direct contact with infected animals or drinking milk.

Human infections are uncommon. A few have been reported in the UK but worldwide distribution is unknown.

The causative agents are *Corynebacterium ulcerans, C. equi, C. pseudotuberculosis, C. pyogenes* (bacterium).

Reservoir and mode of transmission
C. ulcerans has been isolated from humans, horses, cows and monkeys. Human infection may be spread from person to person from contaminated raw milk and from monkey bites. *C. pseudotuberculosis* and *C. pyogenes* have been isolated from sheep, cows, horses and other animals, and human infection occurs when wounds are contaminated by direct contact with animals. *C. equi* is usually identified in horses but the mode of transmission to humans is unclear.

Incubation period
Humans.   Probably 2–5 days.

Animals.   Variable or unknown.

Clinical features
Humans.   *C. ulcerans*: pharyngitis lasting a few days and rarely diphtheria with myocarditis and neurological signs. Bite wound infection. *C. pseudotuberculosis* and *C. pyogenes*: usually infection of wounds and painful regional lymphadenitis which may become chronic. *C. equi* causes prolonged pneumonia in immunosuppressed patients.

Animals.   Abscesses and lymphadenitis, sometimes occurs with *C. pseudotuberculosis*.

Pathology
Humans.   Pharyngitis and tonsilitis with possible pseudo-membrane formation. Pyogenic wound infection.

Animals.   Establish the nature of the infection by culture of lesions and milk.

Special investigations
Humans.   Culture throat swabs, suspect milk and wounds.

Animals.   Culture lesions and milk.

Prognosis
Humans.   Usually mild self-limiting disease.

Animals.   It is a self-limiting disease but recovery may be slow.

Prevention
Humans.   Immunize routinely with diphtheria toxoid which prevents serious disease from other corynebacterial infections.

Animals.   Intramammary infusion of long-acting antibiotic preparations at the end of lactation prevents infection of the udder.

Treatment
Humans. Erythromycin and possibly also diphtheria antitoxin.

Animals. Intramammary infusion of broad-spectrum antibiotics.

Vaccination
Humans. Diphtheria toxoid.

Animals. None.

Legislation
Humans. Clinical diphtheria is notifiable in most countries.

Animals. None.

Cowpox

A rare, benign, virus disease resembling vaccinia virus infection, with lesions of the skin. It is an occupational hazard for milkers. The virus has been isolated only from the UK and western Europe.

The causative agent is cowpox virus (Poxviridae). There is no vaccine.

Reservoir and mode of transmission
The reservoir of infection was believed to be cattle but this is now uncertain. Infection has been recognized in domestic cats in the UK and fatal cases have occured in cheetahs in English zoos. Inapparent infection in a small wild rodent is a suggested reservoir. The virus is transmitted amongst cattle and to milkers by direct contact with skin abrasions.

Incubation period
Humans and animals. 3–7 days.

Clinical features
Humans. The primary lesion at the site of inoculation in the skin develops through macular, papular, vesicular and pustular stages within a few days and is accompanied possibly by fever and lymphadenitis.

Animals.   Mild fever with eruptions on the udder and teats of cattle.

Pathology
Humans.   Papules on the hands and arms develop into vesicles which scab and eventually heal.

Animals.   As for humans, but the vesicles develop on the udder and teats.

Special investigations
Humans.   Identify and isolate virus using electron microscopy of vesicular fluid.

Animals.   Inoculate embryonated eggs to produce haemorrhagic pocks on chicken chorio-allantoic membrane. Stained infected cells contain brick-shaped intracytoplasmic inclusion bodies.

Prognosis
Humans.   It is a mild self-limiting illness.

Animals.   The skin infection is not fatal, but secondary bacterial mastitis is a likely complication.

Prevention
Humans.   Avoid direct contact with infected animals.

Animals.   Impose routine dairy hygiene. Milk affected cows last.

Treatment
Humans and animals.   None.

Legislation
Humans and animals.   None.

Crimean Congo haemorrhagic fever

[Central Asian haemorrhagic fever, Congo fever, tick-borne Crimean Congo haemorrhagic fever]

A tick-borne, viral haemorrhagic fever which occurs in large epidemics, in the Crimean region of the USSR, central Africa, Iraq and Pakistan.

The causative agent is Congo fever virus (Bunyaviridae).

Reservoir and mode of transmission

The reservoir is believed to be cows, goats, hedgehogs, hares, birds and ticks (mainly *Hyalomma* species). Human infection is by the bite of infected adult ticks mainly in agricultural workers in spring and summer during the period of tick activity. Some cases have been associated with contact with raw meat. Person-to-person transmission through contact with blood has been reported. The virus poses a serious hazard to laboratory workers.

Incubation period

Humans.   3–12 days.

Animals.   Not known since the disease is usually subclinical.

Clinical features

Humans.   Illness lasts 3–6 weeks beginning with a sudden onset of fever with headache, pains in arms and legs, anorexia and sometimes vomiting and diarrhoea, flushing of upper body and conjunctivitis. A petechial rash appears within one week and spreads from the upper body, followed by bleeding into skin and from gums and nose, haemoptysis and haematuria.

Animals.   Not known but probably subclinical.

Pathology

Humans.   There is haemorrhage into the skin and various organs.

Animals.   Unknown.

Special investigations

Humans and animals.   Isolate the virus from blood. Serological tests include fluorescent antibody, complement fixation and immunoprecipitin tests.

Prognosis
Humans.   Acute illness usually lasts 1–2 weeks but with prolonged convalescence. The case fatality rate varies from 5 to 50 per cent.

Animals.   Subclinical.

Prevention
Humans.   Control ticks and avoid tick infested areas and tick bites. Avoid inoculation and other exposures in hospitals and laboratories. Apply maximum laboratory safety procedures.

Animals.   Tick control.

Treatment
Humans.   Possibly use convalescent human serum to improve outcome; symptomatic therapy.

Animals.   Inappropriate.

Vaccination
Humans.   May be used in epidemic areas in special circumstances.

Animals.   None.

Legislation
Humans.   Viral haemorrhagic disease is notifiable in some countries, including the UK.

Animals.   None.

Cryptosporidiosis

A recently recognized but common protozoal cause of gastroenteritis, especially in young children worldwide. It can cause life-threatening disease in immunosuppressed patients.

The causative agent is cryptosporidium (Protozoa). There is no vaccine.

Reservoir and mode of transmission
Cryptosporidia have been identified in the faeces of most animal species. Human infection results from person-to-person faecal/oral spread, especially in children, and from raw milk or direct contact with farm animals, especially calves. Water-borne outbreaks have been reported.

Incubation period
Humans and animals. 1–10 days.

Clinical features
Humans. In immunocompetent persons mild mucoid diarrhoea lasts 1–2 weeks, accompanied by vomiting, headache, fever and abdominal pain. In immunocompromised persons there is prolonged, debilitating, profuse, watery diarrhoea with severe weight loss.

Animals. Watery diarrhoea with weight loss occurs in calves.

Pathology
Humans. Nonspecific.

Animals. Atrophy of the villi of the intestine.

Special investigations
Humans and animals. Identify oocysts in faecal smears by special stains.

Prognosis
Humans. Though usually self-limiting it may be life-threatening in immunosuppressed patients, especially those with AIDS.

Animals. Not usually fatal but interrupts growth. Fatality in calves can be high, especially in mixed infections involving other bacterial or viral causes of diarrhoea.

Prevention
Humans. Ensure personal hygiene. Pasteurize milk and ensure adequate filtration of drinking water.

Animals.   Use an all-in/all-out system of calf rearing with rigorous disinfection between batches.

Treatment
Humans.   Symptomatic therapy only.

Animals.   There is no specific therapy. Affected calves must be treated symptomatically with fluid replacement a priority.

Legislation
Humans.   Possibly notifiable when thought to be food-borne infection.

Animals.   None.

Cysticercosis and taeniasis

[Cysticercosis and cysticerciasis refer to infection with the larval stage of *Taenia solium* and *T. saginata*. Taeniasis is infection with the adult tapeworm]

A usually benign tapeworm infection but with a danger of brain damage with the larval stage of *T. solium*. It is acquired by eating undercooked beef or pork and occurs worldwide but especially in Africa and South America.

The causative agents are *Taenia saginata* and *T. solium* in humans, *Cysticercus bovis* in cattle, *C. cellulosae* in pigs and humans (Cestoda). There is no vaccine.

Reservoir and mode of transmission
Pigs and cattle consume ova shed in human faeces. Ova hatch and larvae spread in the circulation to muscles where infective cysts develop. Humans are infected by eating raw or undercooked meat containing larvae. Larvae then mature to adult stage in human intestines. Human cysticercosis occurs when a person (including the original host) ingests *T. solium* eggs passed in human faeces.

Incubation period
Humans.   Cysticercosis: 10–12 days, taeniasis: 8–14 weeks.

Animals. 60 days.

Clinical features
Humans. Tapeworm can cause non-specific abdominal symptoms including anorexia and weight loss. Larval infection produces symptoms attributable to migration through body tissues, such as fever, muscle pains, loss of vision, fits and other neurological symptoms.

Animals. Usually subclinical but signs of muscle pains occur with heavy infestation. Neurological signs may develop.

Pathology
Humans. There is an inflammatory reaction around the larvae.

Animals. In pigs and cattle the cysts in muscle encapsulate with minimal inflammatory reaction. However, myocarditis may occur with heavy infestation and encephalitis if many cysts develop in the brain.

Special investigations
Humans. Examine faeces for eggs or gravid proglottids. Radiological examinations may reveal calcified cysts of *C. cellulosae*.

Animals. Visually examine at meat inspection, but this may fail to detect light infections. Examine muscles, especially heart, masseter and diaphragm muscles for cysts.

Prognosis
Humans. Tapeworm and cyst infections are usually benign, but *C. cellulosae* infection in humans can cause serious, even fatal, brain lesions.

Animals. Cysts usually degenerate in a few months.

Prevention
Humans. Avoid eating raw and undercooked beef or pork. Isolate and treat all patients with *T. solium*. Sanitary disposal of human faeces. Meat inspection to detect animals with cysticercosis.

Animals.   Controlled disposal of sewage.

Treatment
Humans.   Niclosamide, praziquantel. Surgery is sometimes indicated for cysticercosis.

Animals.   None.

Legislation
Humans.   Cystercercosis and taeniasis are notifiable in some countries but not in the UK or the USA.

Animals.   Slaughterhouse legislation in all European Community, and many other, countries requires inspection of meat with incision of muscles in predeliction sites. Carcasses in which cysts are detected may be condemned if infection is heavy, or frozen if infection is light.

Dengue
[Dengue fever, breakbone fever, dengue haemorrhagic fever]

A severe viral fever occurring sporadically and as epidemics transmitted amongst humans and other primates by mosquito bites. It occurs in tropical Asia, the Caribbean, West Africa, Australia, the Pacific islands and Central America.
   The causative agent is Dengue virus (Togaviridae).

Reservoir and mode of transmission
Urban dengue is the result of a man–mosquito cycle of infection. In jungle dengue in South East Asia, primates are thought to be the reservoir of infection. Transmission to humans is by mosquito bite.

Incubation period
Humans.   3–15 days.

Animals.   Unknown.

Clinical features
Humans.   The first phase of illness is usually mild fever, headache, myalgia, lymphadenitis, pharyngitis, rhinitis

and cough lasting 1–5 days and is followed by 1–2 days of remission. The second peak of fever is accompanied by a morbilliform maculopapular rash. Severe haemorrhagic manifestations occur during the second phase with some viruses, especially in children.

Animals.   Probably subclinical.

Pathology
Humans.   Leukopenia and thrombocytopenia occur with haemorrhages in some cases.

Animals.   Unknown.

Special investigations
Humans.   Isolate the virus from blood. Serological tests include complement fixation, haemagglutination inhibition and neutralization tests.

Animals.   Impracticable.

Prognosis
Humans.   The fatality rate of dengue fever in children is low, but may be 10–40 per cent in dengue haemorrhagic fever.

Animals.   Unknown.

Prevention
Humans.   Control mosquitoes and prevent bites. Isolate patients to avoid mosquito bites.

Animals.   Inappropriate.

Treatment
Humans.   Symptomatic therapy.

Animals.   None.

Vaccination
Humans.   Not generally used.

Animals.   None.

Legislation
Humans.   Not notifiable in most countries.

Animals.   None.

Dicroceliosis

[Dicroceliasis, dicrocoeliosis]

A benign, liver disease of herbivores caused by a trematode worm. Humans are accidentally infected by eating ants on raw vegetables. It is widespread in Europe and Asia but has restricted distribution in North America.

The causative agent is *Dicrocoelium dendriticum* (Trematoda). There is no vaccine.

Reservoir and mode of transmission
Herbivores are the definitive hosts. Two intermediate hosts, a snail and an ant, are needed. Eggs are laid in the bile ducts of the definitive hosts. These pass in the bile and faeces. Miracidia hatch and enter the snail. Eventually cercariae emerge in 'slime balls' to be ingested by ants. Infective cysts form in these and herbivores are infected by eating ants on the pasture. Humans are accidental hosts infected by eating ants when nibbling grass or eating fresh vegetables.

Incubation period
Humans.   Uncertain.

Animals.   Unknown.

Clinical features
Humans.   The condition is usually asymptomatic but occasionally there is fever, abdominal discomfort, anorexia and biliary colic. Jaundice is possible.

Animals.   Generally subclinical, but rarely cirrhosis of the liver develops with unthriftyness.

Pathology

Humans. Adult worms localize in bile ducts which become distended and hyperplastic but rarely cirrhotic. Eosinophilia is usual.

Animals. In sheep large numbers of parasites induce cirrhosis. Weight loss, anaemia and oedema occur.

Special investigations

Humans and animals. Identify eggs in faeces and worms in liver biopsy.

Prognosis

Humans. Usually mild or asymptomatic.

Animals. Benign but ill-thrift occurs with heavy infection.

Prevention

Humans. Avoid eating or sucking grass.

Animals. Not attempted.

Treatment

Humans. Praziquantel.

Animals. Not normally required but flukicides may be used for heavy infections.

Legislation

Humans and animals. None.

Dioctophymosis

[Giant kidney worm disease]

A relatively common kidney worm infection of mink and sometimes of dogs and humans caused by eating raw fish. It is found in North and South America, central Europe, Holland, France, Italy, Russia, Japan and Africa, and is especially important in mink in Canada.

The causative agent is *Dioctophyma renale* (Nematoda). There is no vaccine.

Reservoir and mode of transmission
The worm (20–100 cm long) invades the kidney of the definitive host (usually the dog or wild carnivores). Eggs are voided in the urine and probably ingested by an intermediate host, an annelid worm. Larvae in this worm may be eaten by a fish in which they encyst in the muscle. The fish, eaten uncooked by humans or dogs, introduces the infection. The parasite migrates to the kidney to complete the cycle.

Incubation period
Humans and animals.   Uncertain.

Clinical features
Humans.   Renal pain and haematuria may be followed by renal destruction and uraemia.

Animals.   As for humans. Severe weight loss and ill thrift can occur.

Pathology
Humans and animals.   In the few cases reported usually only one worm inhabits one kidney and gradually destroys most of its tissue.

Special investigations
Humans.   Identify eggs in urine.

Animals.   Examine urine sediment for eggs. Laparotomy may be needed to detect peritoneal infections and male worms in the kidney.

Prognosis
Humans.   If untreated, the disease may lead to renal failure and death, but usually only one kidney is involved.

Animals.   Usually subclinical but death from uraemia may occur.

Prevention
Humans.   Avoid eating raw or undercooked fish.

Animals.   Prevent domestic carnivores from eating raw fish.

Treatment
Humans.   Mebendazole. Surgical removal of the kidney is needed in advanced cases.

Animals.   None.

Legislation
Humans and animals.   None.

Diphyllobothriasis

[Fish tapeworm infection]

A benign tapeworm infection of the small intestines caused by eating raw fish.

The causative agents are *Diphyllobothrium latum* and *D. pacificum* (Cestoda). There is no vaccine.

D. latum is common in northern temperate regions where the fish are eaten raw (e.g. in the Baltic countries, Finland and Canada/Alaska). *D. pacificum* is common in coastal South America, especially Peru.

Reservoir and mode of transmission
The definitive hosts of *D. latum* include humans, dogs and cats. For *D. pacificum* the natural reservoir is seals. Two intermediate hosts include a plankton crustacean and a freshwater fish. Gravid proglottids pass in the faeces of the definitive host. The eggs hatch in lakes and waterways and then infect the crustacean. Freshwater fish consume these and the larvae encyst in the musculature. The fish, in their turn, may be eaten by larger fish which can still transmit the infection. Humans acquire the parasite by eating raw infected fish.

Incubation period
Humans.   3–6 weeks from ingestion to adult tapeworm.

Animals. Unknown but presumably as for humans, in dogs and cats.

Clinical features
Humans. The condition is usually asymptomatic. Some patients develop vitamin B_{12} deficiency anaemia. Massive infection may cause diarrhoea and intestinal obstruction.

Animals. No clinical signs are seen in dogs and cats. Heavy infection with larvae can kill the fish intermediate host.

Pathology
Humans. The presence of the large tapeworm, 3 to 10 metres long, in the intestine can cause mechanical obstruction. Megaloblastic anaemia occurs owing to vitamin B_{12} deficiency.

Animals. Subclinical. In fish, myositis and possibly even death occur in heavy infestation.

Special investigations
Humans and animals. Identify characteristic eggs in faeces.

Prognosis
Humans. Usually benign

Animals. Usually benign, but heavy infection may be fatal to fish.

Prevention
Humans and animals. Dispose of faeces hygienically. Educate for proper cooking of fish. Freeze fish or salt cure before marketing.

Treatment
Humans and animals. Anthelmintics, especially niclosamide, quinacrine and praziquantel.

Legislation
Humans and animals. None.

Dipylidiasis

A rare cause of diarrhoea and abdominal pain occurring worldwide, usually in children. It results from infection with a dog or cat tapeworm. Most human cases have been recorded in the USA and Europe.

The causative agent is *Dipylidium caninum* (Cestoda). There is no vaccine.

Reservoir and mode of transmission

Definitive hosts are dogs, cats and their wild counterparts. Intermediate hosts are the fleas, *Ctenocephalides canis* and *C. felis*. Gravid proglottids pass in the faeces of the definitive host. Eggs are released into the environment and are ingested by fleas, in which cysticercoids develop. Dogs and cats are infected by ingesting the infected flea and cysticercoids develop in the gut into adult worms. Humans are accidentally infected by ingesting fleas.

Incubation period

Humans and animals.   Uncertain.

Clinical features

Humans.   Diarrhoea with characteristic gravid proglottids (melon seed shape) appear in faeces. Rarely there is abdominal pain and anal itching.

Animals.   Usually subclinical, though anal irritation is seen rarely.

Pathology

Humans.   Adults worms in small intestine reach 10–80 cm in length.

Animals.   Enteritis occurs rarely in dogs.

Special investigations

Humans and animals.   Identify characteristic mobile proglottids resembling melon seeds in faeces.

Prognosis

Humans and animals.   Usually asymptomatic with no sequelae.

Prevention
Humans.   Control dog and cat fleas with insecticide.

Animals.   Worm dogs and cats regularly and control fleas on dogs and in their surroundings.

Treatment
Humans.   Niclosamide, praziquantel.

Animals.   Control fleas with insecticides. Specific tapeworm remedies include niclosamide.

Legislation
Humans and animals.   None.

Dugbe viral fever

[Nairobi sheep disease (East Africa), ganjam (India)]

A tick-borne viral disease of sheep, cattle and goats, occuring in Nigeria and neighbouring countries, causing fever and dysentery. Humans are occasionally infected in childhood.

The causative agent is Dugbe virus, closely related to Nairobi sheep disease virus (Bunyaviridae).

Reservoir and mode of transmission
Nairobi sheep disease and ganjam viruses cycle between sheep and goats and their ticks; dugbe between cattle and their ticks. Herdsmen and their families are infected by tick bites. Laboratory infections have been reported.

Incubation period
Humans.   4–5 days.

Animals.   4–15 days.

Clinical features
Humans.   Symptoms include fever, rigors, prostration, weakness, lassitude, nausea, vomiting, diarrhoea and possibly a maculopapular rash lasting a few days.

Animals.   Fever, sometimes biphasic, occurs with

depression, weight loss, nasal discharge, dysentery and abortion.

Pathology
Humans. None characteristic.

Animals. There may be enteritis with intestinal haemorrhage; hyperplasia and haemorrhage in lymph nodes:

Special investigations
Humans and animals. Isolate virus from blood. Serological tests include haemagglutination inhibition and complement fixation tests.

Prognosis
Humans. Uncertain.

Animals. In sheep, mortality from Nairobi sheep disease may be 70–90 per cent, but goats are less seriously affected. Dugbe and ganjam are more benign.

Prevention
Humans. Impose strict laboratory safety.

Animals. Qarantine or prohibit imports of live animals from infected countries. Control ticks in enzootic areas.

Treatment
Humans. Symptomatic therapy.

Animals. None.

Vaccination
Humans. None.

Animals. Vaccine can be used to protect animals moving to infected areas.

Legislation
Humans. None.

Animals. Notifiable in some Central American and Caribbean countries.

Echinococcosis

[Hydatid disease, hydatid cyst, hydatidosis]

Infection by the cystic larval form of a canine tapeworm.

The main causative agent is *Echinococcus granulosus*. Other echinococcal species, *E. multilocularis, E. oligarthus* and *E. vogeli*, are less common (Cestoda). There is no vaccine.

E. granulosus is widely distributed in sheep-farming areas throughout the world. *E. multilocularis* is prevalent in Arctic regions but is spreading into eastern and central Europe.

Reservoir and mode of transmission
Sheep form the main intermediate host of *E. granulosus*, but camels, caribou and other ungulates may be intermediate hosts. Dogs, foxes and other canidae are final host reservoirs. Tapeworms in dogs shed eggs which pass in the faeces. Ungulates and humans are infected from dog faeces by the ingestion of eggs which contaminate the environment, dog hairs or vegetables. Dogs are infected by eating raw offal containing the cysts.

The intermediate hosts of *E. multilocularis* are rodents, especially voles, with foxes as the main definitive hosts.

The intermediate host of *E. vogeli* is the paca and the spring rat, with the bush dog as the definitive host.

Incubation period
Humans. Months to many years.

Animals. Eggs are shed in dog faeces from six weeks after infection.

Clinical features
Humans. Symptoms depend on the site of the cyst and its pressure on surrounding tissues. Commonly liver cysts cause abdominal pain and sometimes jaundice. Lung cysts cause chest pain, cough and secondary infection. *E. multilocularis* causes more severe invasive disease. Anaphylactic

shock or secondary bacterial infection may result from rupture of cyst.

Animals. Usually no clinical signs.

Pathology
Humans. This depends on the location of the cysts which, on enlargement, compress the surrounding tissues. An *E. granulosus* cyst consists of an inner germinal layer which may bud to form daughter cysts which can spread widely if the parent cyst ruptures. The outer laminated wall of cyst may calcify and the cyst remain asymptomatic. In *E. multilocularis* there is not a substantial outer wall and cysts aggressively invade tissues.

Animals. No lesions occur in dogs which harbour the tapeworm (except for enteritis in heavy infestations), but the hydatid cysts in sheep cause considerable condemnation of meat and loss of production.

Special investigations
Humans. Localize carcass cysts by X-ray, ultrasound and other imaging techniques. The Casoni skin test is unreliable. Serological test include complement fixation, ELISA, latex agglutination and immunodiffusion tests.

Animals. Purge dogs and examine faeces for tapeworms. Serological tests are being developed for intermediate hosts.

Prognosis
Humans. This varies with the site and activity of cysts. There is high fatality from *E. multilocularis* and from cerebral cysts of *E. granulosus*.

Animals. Subclinical in intermediate and final hosts.

Prevention
Humans. Wash hands after handling dogs, avoid dog faeces and prevent dogs soiling the immediate environment, vegetables etc. Apply laboratory safety precautions when handling worms and eggs.

Animals. Systematically and regularly worm dogs to eradicate infection. Prevent dogs scavenging carcasses and raw offal. Bury sheep carcasses.

Treatment
Humans. Surgically remove cysts. Mebendazole and albendazole may be useful.

Animals. Worm dogs using an anthelmintic effective against tapeworms (e.g. praziquantel).

Legislation
Humans. The condition is notifiable in some countries, including Australia, New Zealand and some European countries.

Animals. Slaughterhouse and waste food legislation in some countries requires sterilization of infected offal. Compulsory burial of sheep carcasses and exclusion of dogs from abattoirs is required in the UK where meat inspection legislation requires condemnation of affected organs. The disease is notifiable in cattle and sheep in some Central and South American and European countries, Cyprus, New Zealand, and New Guinea.

Echinostomiasis

[Echinostomatidosis]

A relatively mild worm infection caused by eating under-cooked snails, mainly in India, China, South East Asia and the East Indies.

The causative agents are species of *Echinostoma* (Trematoda). There is no vaccine.

Reservoir and mode of transmission
Definitive hosts include a wide variety of wild and domestic animals and some birds in addition to humans. Two inter-mediate hosts include a snail and another mollusc or a fish. Humans and other definitive hosts are infected on eating undercooked snails.

Incubation period
Humans and animals.   Uncertain.

Clinical features
Humans.   It is often asymptomatic but abdominal pain and diarrhoea occasionally occur.

Animals.   Usually mild or subclinical.

Pathology
Humans and animals.   Mild enteritis and even ulceration are possible.

Special investigations
Humans and animals.   Identify eggs in faeces.

Prognosis
Humans.   It is usually asymptomatic, or there may be mild symptoms with no sequelae.

Animals.   A benign infection.

Prevention
Humans.   Avoid eating raw snails.

Animals.   Avoid feeding raw fish to domestic animals.

Treatment
Humans.   Praziquantel.

Animals.   None.

Legislation
Humans and animals.   None.

Epidemic polyarthritis

[Murray valley rash, Ross River disease, Ross River fever, arthropod-borne viral arthritis and rash, epidemic polyarthritis and rash]

A febrile viral disease associated with a skin rash and inflammation of joints. It is transmitted by mosquito bite from wild animals, in Australia, New Guinea, Fiji and American Samoa.

The causative agent is Ross River virus (Togaviridae). There is no vaccine.

Reservoir and mode of transmission
Infection is widespread in animals including wallabies as well as mosquitoes which transmit infection to humans by bite.

Incubation period
Humans.   About 10 days.

Animals.   Unknown.

Clinical features
Humans.   There is mild fever, sore throat, pain and swelling in joints, especially those of the hands and feet, lasting up to two weeks. A maculopapular rash may be present.

Animals.   Unknown.

Pathology
Humans.   Inflammation of joints.

Animals.   Unknown.

Special investigations
Humans and animals. Serological tests include haemagglutination inhibition and complement fixation tests; rarely, isolation of virus from blood.

Prognosis
Humans.   This is a self-limiting disease but prolonged arthritis is possible.

Animals.   Unknown.

Prevention
Humans.   Control vector mosquitoes and prevent their bites.

Animals. Inappropriate.

Treatment
Humans. Symptomatic therapy.

Animals. Inapplicable.

Legislation
Humans. Notifiable in New Zealand.

Animals. None.

Equine encephalitis

[Eastern equine encephalomyelitis, western equine encephalitis, eastern, western and Venezuelan encephalitis]

A group of febrile viral diseases of horses and humans frequently leading to fatal encephalitis. It is transmitted by mosquitoes from wildlife reservoirs and occurs sporadically and in epidemics usually in summer and autumn.

Eastern encephalitis (EEE) occurs in coastal regions of the eastern states of Canada and North and Central America, Trinidad, Guyana, Brazil and Argentina. Western encephalitis (WEE) occurs in North America, Mexico, Guyana, Brazil and Argentina. Venezuelan encephalitis (VEE) occurs in Venezuela, Colombia, Central and South America.

The causative agents are the equine encephalitis group of viruses (Togaviridae).

Reservoir and mode of transmission

The reservoir of infection is mosquitoes and wild birds (EEE and WEE) or small rodents and marsupials (VEE). The viruses cycle naturally between their wild bird or animal hosts and a wide variety of mosquito species. Horses, mules, donkeys, pheasants and man are accidental hosts infected by mosquito bites and probably play no part in the transmission cycles. Infection from laboratory accidents has occurred.

Incubation period

Humans and animals. 1–3 weeks.

Clinical features

Humans.   Fever begins suddenly with severe headache, sore throat and conjunctivitis followed 1–2 days later by delirium, convulsions and paralysis. Fever may be biphasic in children followed by fatal encephalitis within five days.

Animals.   Of the many hosts only the horse shows clear clinical signs. These are peracute with sudden onset of high fever progressing rapidly to death in most cases. Longer-term survivors show signs of encephalitis with tremors, paralysis etc.

Pathology

Humans.   Extensive necrosis involves large areas of the midbrain. Neutrophil infiltration with perivascular cuffing and gliosis is characteristic.

Animals.   Haemorrhages and degeneration of neurones occur throughout the brain. Eventually perivascular cuffing and gliosis occur.

Special investigations

Humans and animals.   Isolate virus from the brain at necropsy. Serological tests include complement fixation, haemagglutination inhibition and neutralization tests.

Prognosis

Humans.   The fatality rate in humans for EEE is up to 80 per cent and for WEE 3–15 per cent. VEE is less severe, but as with EEE and WEE there is long-term disability in survivors with mental retardation of children, paralysis and convulsions.

Animals.   There is 90 per cent fatality rate amongst horses, in outbreaks.

Prevention

Humans.   Control mosquitoes and prevent their bites. Apply strict laboratory safety procedures.

Animals.   As above, and vaccinate horses where disease risk exists. Stable horses during outbreaks.

Treatment
Humans.   Symptomatic therapy.

Animals.   Supportive therapy.

Vaccination
Humans.   Possibly use inactivated freeze-dried EEE and WEE vaccines for persons with extensive occupational exposure.

Animals.   Horses may be vaccinated annually in the spring using inactivated chick embryo vaccines against EEE and WEE which may be combined.

Legislation
Humans.   Acute encephalitis is notifiable in many countries, including the UK and the USA.

Animals.   In Great Britain and some other countries, there is notification, quarantine and prohibition of imports from infected countries. There are official control schemes in Mexico, Nicaragua and the Dominican Republic. There is a slaughter policy in Norway, West Germany and Japan.

Erlichiosis

[Ehrlichiosis, tick-borne fever]

A newly recognized and poorly understood tick-borne rickettsial infection. It occurs worldwide in dogs, and in other animals in Great Britain, Scandinavia and India.
   The causative agent is *Ehrlichia canis* (rickettsia). There is no vaccine.

Reservoir and mode of transmission
Dogs and the brown dog tick (*Rhipicephalus sanguineus*) form the natural reservoir. It is presumably transmitted to humans by tick bite. In Europe, sheep and *Ixodes ricinus* ticks are involved and *Rhipicephalus sanguineus* in India.

Incubation period
Humans.   Uncertain, possibly about ten days.

Animals.   Unknown.

Clinical features
Humans.   The few reported cases have had fever, rigors, myalgia, headache, nausea, anorexia and sometimes uraemia, haematuria, encephalopathy, hepatitis, thrombocytopenia and anaemia.

Animals.   Uncertain.

Pathology
Humans.   Unclear, but most reported cases had leucopenia and thrombocytopenia.

Animals.   Unclear.

Special investigations
Humans and animals.   Stain blood smears to demonstrate the parasites in neutrophils and monocytes. The indirect fluorescent antibody test has been used.

Prognosis
Humans.   Unclear.

Animals.   There is subclinical or only mild fever in sheep, cattle and goats. Young animals are less susceptible. Abortions occur in newly infected herds and flocks. Infection decreases resistance to other tick-borne diseases.

Prevention
Humans.   Avoid tick bites. Control vector ticks.

Animals.   Control ticks in sheep by dipping or spraying using insecticide suspensions.

Treatment
Humans.   Tetracyclines.

Animals.   Ethoxyethylglyoxal dithiosemicarbazone is the drug of choice. Sulphadimidine is effective in sheep but relapses may occur.

Legislation
Humans. All rickettsial infections are notifiable in a few countries such as France and Israel.
Animals. None.

Erysipeloid

[Erysipelas, diamonds (in pigs)]

A bacterial skin infection of pig handlers, abattoir workers and fish workers, worldwide. It is associated with arthritis.

The causative agent is *Erysipelothrix rhusiopathiae* (bacterium).

Reservoir and mode of transmission
The organism is common in animals and in soil. Human infection is acquired when the organism contaminates cuts and abrasions, usually on the hand or forearm.

Incubation period
Humans and animals. 2–7 days.

Clinical features
Humans. Localized erythema occurs with pain and oedema of skin spreading peripherally. Arthritis may develop in finger joints. Rarely it causes generalized infection and septicaemia.

Animals. In its acute form the disease begins as a high fever with later development of characteristic diamond-shaped lesions on the skin. The chronic form shows painful enlarged joints and eventually signs of heart disease.

Pathology
Humans. Non-specific skin lesions and arthritis.

Animals. Arthritis and endocarditis with vegetations on heart valves occur.

Special investigations
Humans and animals. Isolate the organism from the skin lesion or blood.

Prognosis
Humans.   Fatality is rare in humans and the disease usually remains a mild skin inflammation.

Animals.   In pigs untreated cases often progress to the chronic stage with variable mortality and debility.

Prevention
Humans.   Ensure good hygiene. Wash hands and use gloves and wound dressings where applicable.

Animals.   Keep pigs on concrete. Vaccinate either at 6–10 weeks of age, or 10–12 weeks where sows are routinely vaccinated, with a booster 2–4 weeks later. Sows should be vaccinated twice yearly, 3–6 weeks before farrowing.

Treatment
Humans.   Penicillin and erythromycin.

Animals.   Responds well to penicillin by injection, often given with erysipelas antiserum.

Vaccination
Humans.   None.

Animals.   Vaccination, used in pigs and turkeys where infection is enzootic, provides six months immunity but is not uniformly effective against all strains of the organism.

Legislation
Humans.   Occupationally acquired infection may be notifiable in some countries.

Animals.   Notifiable in some countries of all continents except North America and Australasia. Slaughter policy exists in Cuba, USSR, Albania and Japan.

Esophagostomiasis

[Nodular intestinal worm infection, oesophagostomiasis]

An intestinal worm infection of primates transmitted by the

faecal–oral route. It occurs mainly in Africa, but occasionally in South America and Asia.

The causative agents are *Oesphagostomum stephanostomum*, *O. bifurcum* and *O. aculeatum* (Nematoda). There is no vaccine.

Reservoir and mode of transmission
The parasite lives in the intestines of various primates and sometimes in humans. These definitive hosts can also serve as intermediate hosts. Eggs passed in faeces release larvae which infect the definitive host on ingestion. The parasite invades the intestinal wall to form nodules. The fourth stage larvae which develop in these nodules migrate to the lumen of the large intestine to form the adult worm and complete the cycle.

Incubation period
Humans and animals. Uncertain.

Clinical features
Humans. Mild infection goes unnoticed but sometimes abdominal pain, and gastrointestinal bleeding and even peritonitis occur.

Animals. Mild infection is subclinical. Abdominal pain follows more severe infection with diarrhoea or even dysentery.

Pathology
Humans. Granulomatous nodules in the intestinal wall contain larvae and parasites. These may be secondarily infected and lead to abscesses.

Animals. As for humans. Death in the non-human primates may ensue from perforation of the intestine and peritonitis.

Special investigations
Humans and animals. Identify worm eggs in faeces. Culture to obtain larvae for species identification.

Prognosis

Humans and animals. This varies from asymptomatic infection to dysenteric disease or even fatal peritonitis.

Prevention

Humans. Ensure good personal hygiene. Sanitary disposal of faeces is important.

Animals. Ensure routine hygiene in laboratory primates.

Treatment

Humans. Anthelmintic therapy.

Animals. Anthelmintic therapy may be attempted in laboratory primates.

Legislation

Humans and animals. None.

Fascioliasis

[Liver fluke disease]

A fluke infection of the liver, mainly of sheep and cattle, which can progress to severe cirrhosis. Humans are rare accidental hosts.

The causative agents are *Fasciola hepatica* and *F. gigantica* (Trematoda). There is no vaccine.

In animals *F. hepatica* is distributed worldwide, whilst *F. gigantica* is most common in Africa, India and southern USA. Human infections have been reported in sheep and cattle farming areas of South America, the West Indies, Europe, Australia and the Middle East.

Reservoir and mode of transmission

Domestic and wild herbivores are the principal hosts and reservoirs. Adult parasites in the bile ducts lay eggs which pass into the faeces. On hatching the miracidium enters the intermediate host which is usually a snail, *Lymnaea truncatula*. Cercariae leave the snail and encyst on plant leaves especially near stagnant water (e.g. on watercress). Animals and humans are infected if they eat (or nibble) these infected leaves. Larvae are released in the duodenum and migrate to the liver to complete the life-cycle.

Incubation period
Humans and animals. Variable.

Clinical features
Humans. The severity of symptoms depends on the number of flukes. These may be fever, rigors, abdominal pain, jaundice and tender liver. Subcutaneous inflamed tracks can be caused by migrating larvae.

Animals. Loss of production, wasting and sometimes anaemia with jaundice and death may occur. Animals become susceptible to metabolic disorders such as ketosis.

Pathology
Humans. Hepatomegaly and eosinophilia occur. Heavy infestation causes cholangitis, biliary cirrhosis and cholelithiasis. Migration of the parasite produces tracts of traumatic necrosis and micro-abscesses.

Animals. As for humans. Chronic cirrhosis (pipestem liver) is common in sheep.

Special investigations
Humans. Identify eggs in faeces or bile aspirate. Perform a liver biopsy. Serological tests include complement fixation, indirect haemagglutination and electrophoresis tests.

Animals. Examine faeces for characteristic eggs.

Prognosis
Humans. The condition is usually self-limiting, but recurrent biliary obstruction and secondary infection may lead to chronic liver damage.

Animals. Acute fascioliasis, due to migration of immature flukes, can be rapidly fatal with high mortality in young sheep. Large numbers of adult flukes in the bile ducts cause chronic wasting in sheep and cattle.

Prevention
Humans. Do not grow watercress in water accessible to herbivores and their faeces.

Animals. In high-risk areas treat sheep and cattle in late autumn and spring. In the UK the degree of risk and best time to treat are forecast from meteorological data. Apply molluscicides to wet areas in spring or early summer. Keep sheep and cattle away from wet areas in autumn and winter. Control hares and rabbits which may harbour the parasite.

Treatment
Humans. Praziquantel.

Animals. Rafoxanide, brotianide, clioxanide and nichlopholan by mouth are effective against mature and immature *F. hepatica*. Rafoxanide is also known to be active against *F. gigantica*. Nitroxynil by subcutaneous injection is effective in cattle.

Legislation
Humans. None.

Animals. Notifiable in cattle and sheep in some Central and South American countries, Italy and Czechoslovakia.

Filariasis

[Filariosis, brugiasis]

A mosquito-borne roundworm infection which is only occasionally zoonotic. It can induce gross enlargement and deformity of limbs.

The commonest causative agent is *Wuchererioa bancrofti*, which is not zoonotic. *Brugei malayi* is zoonotic. *Dirofilaria immitis* may occasionally infect humans (Nematoda). There is no vaccine.

The zoonotic form, *B. malayi*, has been identified in Malaya and the Philippines. *D. immitis* occurs in dogs in North and South America, Australia, India, the Far East and Europe; but human infections have been reported mainly from the USA, with a few from Canada and Australia.

Reservoir and mode of transmission
Certain wild animals (monkeys and felines) are the reservoirs for *B. malayi*, but dogs carry *D. immitis*, humans

being only an aberrant host. Transmission to humans is via the bite of a mosquito vector (Mansonia and Anopheles). These, on biting humans, release microfilariae on to skin which enter the body through the puncture wound and pass via the lymphatics to lymph nodes. The worms are viviparous, producing microfilariae. These appear in the blood and reinfect the biting insect.

Incubation period
Humans. 3–15 months.

Animals. Variable, but several months.

Clinical features
Humans. Repeated bouts of fever, lymphadenopathy, lymphangitis and abscesses occur. Gross enlargement of limbs (elephantiasis) and rarely hydrocele may progress over years.

Animals. *D. immitis* is found in the right ventricle of dogs and in the pulmonary artery. Mild infection causes no signs, but long continued infection leads to cardiac insufficiency with ascites and passive congestion.

Pathology
Humans. Eosinophilia. The main lesions are lymphangitis and lymphadenitis. This leads to lymphatic obstruction and massive lymphoedema followed by fibrosis (so-called elephantiasis) especially in the legs. Pulmonary nodules have been reported.

Animals. The lesions are not known except for *D. immitis* in dogs, and these are generally endocarditis and arteritis with thrombosis.

Special investigations
Humans and animals. Identify microfilariae in blood. Serological tests incluse ELISA, indirect immunofluorescence and indirect haemagglutination tests.

Prognosis
Humans. The clinical course is highly variable, but

elephantiasis is not easily reversible.

Animals.   Most infections are subclinical or mild.

Prevention
Humans.   Control vectors and avoid their bites.

Animals.   Treat dogs with thiacetarsamide every six months in highly enzootic areas.

Treatment
Humans.   Diethylcarbamazine is effective but may provoke allergic reactions, which can be controlled by antihistamines.

Animals.   Inappropriate.

Legislation
Humans and animals.   None.

Flea-borne typhus fever

[Murine typhus, endemic typhus fever, urban typhus]

A febrile rickettsial disease transmitted by rat fleas, worldwide but especially in warmer regions.
     The causative agent is *Rickettsia typhi* (rickettsia). There is no vaccine.

Reservoir and mode of transmission
Rats are the main reservoir and their fleas are the main vector (*Xenopsylla cheopis*). Humans are infected by contamination of flea bites, broken skin or conjunctivae by flea faeces. Domestic animals may transport the flea vector to humans. Inhalation of contaminated dust may be a route of infection.

Incubation period
Humans.   5–23 days.

Animals.   Unknown.

Clinical features
Humans. There is a gradual onset of fever with severe headache, rigors, generalized pains and dry cough (sometimes developing to bronchopneumonia) of about two weeks' duration. A macular rash appears by about five days, first appearing on the trunk and lasting about six days. CNS manifestations are possible.

Animals. Unknown, but probably subclinical.

Pathology
Humans. Damage is caused to vascular endothelia by invasion of rickettsia, possibly leading to thrombosis and haemorrhage.

Animals. The agent localizes in the brain and various organs but with no known lesions.

Special investigations
Humans. Isolate the organism from blood using guinea pigs or embryonated eggs. Serological tests include Weil-Felix, complement fixation and indirect fluorescent antibody tests.

Animals. Rarely attempted, but as for humans.

Prognosis
Humans. The fatality rate in untreated cases is about 1–2 per cent.

Animals. Subclinical.

Prevention
Humans. Control rat fleas with residual insecticides followed by control of rodents.

Animals. Impracticable.

Treatment
Humans. Tetracyclines and chloramphenicol.

Animals. Inappropriate.

Legislation
Humans. Typhus (all forms) is notifiable in many countries, including Australia, New Zealand and the UK.

Animals. None.

Foot and mouth disease

[Aphthus fever, aphthosis]

An acute, highly infectious, viral disease of cloven-footed animals with very rare spread to humans. It is enzootic in Africa, Asia and Europe. The North American and Australasian continents are free from disease. In some countries, including the UK, eradication is maintained by vigorous control measures, but infection is introduced from abroad occasionally.

The causative agent is the foot and mouth disease virus (Picornaviridae).

Reservoir and mode of transmission
Wild ruminants provide the reservoir of infection for domestic animals. The route of infection is by inhalation and ingestion. Wind plays an important part in local spread and waste food in international spread. Infected animals excrete virus in all secretions and excretions from shortly before the appearance of vesicles. The virus persists for weeks on premises, clothing and equipment, and indefinitely in frozen meat where it survives in lymph nodes, bone marrow and offal in which pH changes are minimal.

Incubation period
Humans. Uncertain.

Animals. 1–21 but usually 3–8 days.

Clinical features
Humans. The disease is nearly always subclinical, but with survival of virus in the pharynx and tonsil for up to two weeks. There may be fever with vesicles on lips, in the mouth and on the hands and feet for a few days.

Animals. Biungulates show fever, anorexia, profuse salivation and lameness. Vesicles form on the coronary band of the feet and in the mouth, tongue and lips.

Pathology
Humans and animals. Virus penetrates the mucosa and forms a primary vesicle. Viraemia follows many secondary vesicles, which burst leaving large red erosions. Sometimes lesions spread to organs such as the heart, which undergoes degeneration of the myocardium.

Special investigations
Humans. Isolate virus from lesions.

Animals. Serology. Virus can be isolated in tissue culture and in suckling mice. Because of the importance of this disease calf inoculation may be used to differentiate it from other vesicular diseases.

Prognosis
Humans. It is a mild self-limiting infection with full recovery in 1–2 weeks.

Animals. Variations in virulence occur, but mortality is usually low where the disease runs its course.

Prevention
Humans. Not considered necessary.

Animals. Prohibit importation of animals and animal products from countries where disease occurs. Vaccinate susceptible animals in a buffer zone between infected and clean areas. Slaughter infected animals and their contacts when outbreaks occur in non-enzootic areas.

Treatment
Humans and animals. None.

Vaccination
Humans. None.

Animals. Regular vaccination is practised in many

countries of South America, Africa, Europe and Asia using killed multivalent vaccines against the strains prevalent in the region. Because of the risks of masking infection and confusing serological tests, vaccination is prohibited in countries in which disease has been eradicated.

Legislation
Humans.   None.

Animals.   Notifiable with slaughter policy in many countries.

Gastrodiscoidiasis

[Amphistomiasis]

A flatworm infection of the caecum, occasionally causing diarrhoea. It is acquired by ingesting eggs on aquatic leaves, in India, Malaysia and South East Asia.

The causative agent is *Gastrodiscoides* (*Amphistomum*) *hominis* (Trematoda). There is no vaccine.

Reservoir and mode of transmission
Worms inhabit the large intestine of the definitive host, including humans, pigs (in India) and the mouse deer (*Tragulus napin*) in Malaysia. The eggs pass in the faeces. Miracidia hatch and infect a snail (*Helicorbis coenosus*) which may be the intermediate host. Cercariae emerge and encyst on aquatic plants and humans are infected by eating the leaves.

Incubation period
Humans.   Uncertain.

Animals.   Unknown.

Clinical features
Humans and animals.   The condition is usually subclinical, but abdominal discomfort and diarrhoea with heavy infestation may occur.

Pathology
Humans and animals. Worms attach to mucosa of caecum and ascending colon, producing local inflammation.

Special investigations
Humans and animals. Identify eggs in faeces.

Prognosis
Humans. The disease is usually asymptomatic, unless there is heavy infestation.

Animals. Subclinical or mild transient illness.

Prevention
Humans. Ensure good personal hygiene and sanitary disposal of faeces.

Animals. Prevent pigs from eating aquatic plants.

Treatment
Humans. Praziquantel and tetrachlorethylene are used.

Animals. None attempted.

Legislation
Humans and animals. None.

Giardiasis

[Lambliasis, giardia enteritis]

A mild, protozoal enteritis usually acquired by the human faecal–oral route, but occasionally from water contaminated by animal faeces. It occurs worldwide, especially in areas of poor sanitation.

The causative agent is *Giardia lamblia* (Protozoa). There is no vaccine.

Reservoir and mode of transmission
Humans are the main reservoir, with transmission by faecal–oral spread especially in young children in nurseries. Animal reservoirs, especially the beaver and muskrat in

North America, may contaminate drinking water supplies to cause large water-borne outbreaks.

Incubation period
Humans.   1–4 weeks.

Animals.   Unknown.

Clinical features
Humans.   There is intermittent abdominal pain and distension, flatulence, and prolonged or intermittent diarrhoea and steatorrhoea, with weight loss. Malabsorption can last for several weeks.

Animals.   It is usually subclinical but can cause malabsortion diarrhoea and weight loss in dogs and cats. In caged birds there is anorexia and emaciation during which diarrhoea occurs with loose light-coloured droppings. Death follows eventually.

Pathology
Humans.   Enterocyte damage occurs only in severe cases.

Animals.   Occasionally there is villous atrophy in the small intestine.

Special investigations
Humans.   Identify cysts or trophozoites in faecal smears or biopsies from the small intestine.

Animals.   Examine faeces for the parasite.

Prognosis
Humans and animals.   The illness is self-limiting, with complete recovery.

Prevention
Humans.   Ensure good personal hygiene and sanitary disposal of faeces. Filtrate and chlorinate drinking water, and boil water to destroy cysts.

Animals. Ensure sanitary disposal of sewage and good processing of sewage effluent.

Treatment
Humans. Metronidazole.

Animals. Inappropriate.

Legislation
Humans. Not usually notifiable.

Animals. None.

Glanders

[Farcy]

A rare, potentially fatal, bacterial disease transmitted from infected horses. Once common worldwide but now eradicated from many countries, it is still seen in Asia, North Africa, eastern Europe and Asia, especially Mongolia.

The causative agent is *Pseudomonas mallei* (bacterium). There is no vaccine.

Reservoir and mode of transmission
Horses, mules and donkeys are the main reservoir. Transmission between animals is by ingestion or inhalation of infected nasal discharges which contaminate the environment. Cats and dogs may be infected from contaminated horse meat. Human infection is by contamination of wounds by close contact with infected horses or carcasses, or laboratory accidents.

Incubation period
Humans. 1–14 days.

Animals. Days to months.

Clinical features
Humans. Initially there is fever, malaise and muscle and joint pains often leading to pneumonia, pleurisy and pyaemia. There is cellulitis with painful nodules in the skin, and nasal mucosa, with a foul discharge. Untreated disease progresses to death within three weeks in most cases,

although a chronic form may occur in which there is abscess formation in skin, joints and muscle.

Animals.   The acute form involves fever, dyspnoea, diarrhoea and rapid loss of weight with eventual death. The chronic form gives slowly progressing respiratory distress with coughing, and a nasal discharge. Nodules with suppuration may affect the skin (farcy).

Pathology
Humans.   Characteristic nodules and abscesses occur in lungs, liver, spleen and skin.

Animals.   Fibrous nodules occur in the lungs, which eventually caseate and calcify. In the nasal cavities ulceration results in a mucopurulent discharge. The cutaneous lesions begin as fibrous nodules which suppurate.

Special investigations
Humans.   Isolate the causal agent by inoculation of hamsters. Various tests available include the mallein skin test, complement fixation and haemagglutination tests.

Animals.   Isolate the organism by culture or laboratory animal inoculation (guinea pigs, hamster). The mallein test diagnoses latent and chronic infection in the horse. It involves inoculating 0.1 ml of concentrated whole culture (mallein) into the eyelid. Oedematous swelling, conjunctival congestion and mucoid discharge indicate a positive reaction. Serological tests are also available.

Prognosis
Humans.   The fatality rate is about 95 per cent in untreated cases.

Animals.   Horses usually suffer chronic and sometimes fatal illness. Asses and mules usually suffer acute disease which is often fatal.

Prevention
Humans.   Eradicate equine infection. Ensure strict hygiene when handling infected animals. Laboratory safety is especially important.

Animals. Detect infected horses and disinfect all stables and equipment. Prohibit imports from countries where disease still occurs. Quarantine and mallein test all animals on import or export. Destroy affected animals, mallein test contacts and destroy reactors. Disinfect grooming and feeding equipment and surroundings.

Treatment
Humans. Antibiotic therapy.

Animals. Inappropriate.

Legislation
Humans. The condition is not usually notifiable.

Animals. This is a notifiable disease with slaughter policy in many countries, including Great Britain.

Group C bunyaviral fever

[Marituba fever, Caraparu fever]

A benign, febrile, viral disease of forest workers in South America, transmitted from wild animals by mosquitoes.

The causative agents are the group C bunyaviruses (Bunyaviridae). There is no vaccine.

Reservoir and mode of transmission
Viruses have been isolated from various wild animals, including rodents and monkeys. Transmission is by mosquito bite.

Incubation period
Humans. 3–12 days.

Animals. Unknown.

Clinical features
Humans. There is fever, severe headache and influenza-like symptoms, with prostration for a few days and possibly a prolonged convalescence.

Animals. Usually subclinical.

Pathology
Humans.   None characteristic.

Animals.   None.

Special investigations
Humans and animals.   Isolate virus from blood by animal inoculation. Serological tests include a complement fixation test.

Prognosis
Humans and animals.   It is usually a benign self-limiting illness.

Prevention
Humans.   Avoid mosquito-infested areas and mosquito bites.

Animals.   None.

Treatment
Humans.   Symptomatic therapy.

Animals.   None.

Legislation
Humans and animals.   None.

Haemorrhagic colitis

[Haemolytic uraemic syndrome (HUS)]

A newly recognized, bacterial, enteric, food-borne disease which may lead to haemolytic anaemia with renal failure. The geographical distribution is probably worldwide.

The causative agents are verotoxin-producing strains of *Escherichia coli*. Serogroup 0157:H7 is most commonly implicated. There is no vaccine.

Reservoir and mode of transmission

Cattle have been identified as a reservoir of infection for humans. The disease is a food-borne infection, especially via undercooked beef and raw milk and by person-to-person faecal–oral spread.

Incubation period
Humans. Probably 1–12 days.

Animals. Uncertain.

Clinical features
Humans. Symptoms range from mild diarrhoea to severe abdominal pain with profuse watery or bloody diarrhoea with or without low-grade fever but of short duration. Haemorrhagic diarrhoea may be followed by haemolysis and renal failure.

Animals. Disease specifically associated with human pathogenic strains has not yet been characterized, but *E. coli* can cause diarrhoea in calves and mastitis in cows, often accompanied by toxaemia.

Pathology
Humans. There is inflammation and haemorrhage of the intestinal wall, with dilation and oedema of caecum and colon. HUS is characterized by haemolysis, thrombocytopenia and renal failure.

Animals. Septicaemic forms of *E. coli* disease induce widespread petechial haemorrhages with occasional meningitis and arthritis.

Special investigations
Humans and animals. Isolate and serotype the causal organism from faeces, and identify verotoxins in faeces by DNA probes.

Prognosis
Humans. Haemorrhagic colitis is usually a self-limiting disease of less than seven days, but severe haemorrhage and death have been reported. HUS may lead to chronic renal failure in a high proportion of cases.

Animals.   Severe diarrhoea may lead to dehydration and death.

Prevention
Humans.   Heat-treat milk. Thoroughly cook meat. Ensure good food and personal hygiene.

Animals.   Total prevention of *E. coli* infection is impossible. Keep young animals in small groups in warm, comfortable, clean surroundings; ensure adequate colostrum intake; avoid abrupt changes in feeding; isolate scouring animals; depopulate, clean, disinfect and rest buildings between batches of calves.

Treatment
Humans.   This is supportive, including renal dialysis. Antibiotic therapy may be indicated.

Animals.   Oral antibiotics and fluid replacement.

Legislation
Humans.   The condition is notifiable in many countries if due to food-poisoning.

Animals.   None.

Haemorrhagic fever with renal syndrome

[Korean haemorrhagic fever, nephropathia epidemica, epidemic haemorrhagic fever, haemorrhagic nephrosonephritis]

A severe, febrile, haemorrhagic, viral disease transmitted by rodents and capable of causing kidney failure. It occurs sporadically and in outbreaks. The geographical distribution is not completely delineated, but the disease is well-documented in Asia, USSR, Japan, Northern Europe and the USA. It was first recognized during the Korean war in 1951.

The causative agent is Hantaan virus (Bunyaviridae). There is no vaccine.

Reservoir and mode of transmission

The reservoir is wild rodents, including house rats, which excrete virus in urine and saliva. The mode of transmission is not clearly defined but it is not transmitted from person to person. Laboratory animals may be a source of human infection and laboratory accidents have occurred.

Incubation period

Humans. 1–5 weeks.

Animals. Unknown.

Clinical features

Humans. Symptoms begin with the sudden onset of fever which lasts 1–2 weeks, accompanied by prostration, anorexia, generalized pains, conjunctivitis, proteinuria and hypotension, possibly followed by haemorrhages and haematuria with renal failure.

Animals. Subclinical.

Pathology

Humans. Congestion and haemorrhages are seen in the kidneys and other organs.

Animals. None.

Special investigations

Humans. Serological tests include the fluorescent antibody test.

Animals. None.

Prognosis

Humans. The fatality rate is about 5 per cent, although more severe disease is seen in the Far East than in Scandinavia.

Animals. Subclinical.

Prevention
Humans.   Control rodents. Apply strict laboratory safety procedures.

Animals.   None.

Treatment
Humans.   None except supportive therapy.

Animals.   None.

Legislation
Humans.   The disease is notifiable in South Korea. Viral haemorrhagic disease is notifiable in the UK.

Animals.   None.

Herpes virus simiae infection

[Simian B disease, B virus infection]

A viral skin infection from monkeys, capable of progression to a fatal encephalitis. Laboratory exposure to Old World monkeys is the main human hazard. It occurs in Asia and Africa where enzootic in monkeys.

The causative agent is herpes virus simiae (Herpes viridae).

Reservoir and mode of transmission
Primates of the Macaca genus, chiefly the rhesus monkey (*M. mulatta*), are the reservoir. Transmission amongst monkeys is by direct contact, bites and scratches, contamination of food and water by saliva and possibly by aerosol. Humans are infected by bites and scratches and contamination of abraded skin by monkey saliva. Human-to-human transmission is not known to occur. The virus poses a serious hazard to laboratory workers.

Incubation period
Humans.   1–5 weeks.

Animals.   Unknown, but probably as for humans.

Clinical features
Humans. Symptoms include fever, headache, muscle pains, vertigo, abdominal pain and finally ascending flaccid paralysis and death within three weeks in most cases.

Animals. Small and inconspicuous vesicles in the mouth.

Pathology
Humans. A vesicle appears at the point of entry, followed by lymphadenitis. Encephalitis is seen with necrotic foci in the viscera.

Animals. The initial vesicle breaks down to leave a small ulcer which heals rapidly.

Special investigations
Humans. Isolate virus from the brain at necropsy. Serological tests include immunofluorescence and serum neutralization tests.

Animals. Inspect the mouth and tongue of anaesthetized monkeys for vesicles and diphtheritic ulcers; serology.

Prognosis
Humans. The condition is usually fatal once clinically affected and survivors may have permanent brain damage.

Animals. There is benign and transient infection in monkeys.

Prevention
Humans. Quarantine recently imported monkeys for 6–8 weeks and destroy any which show lesions. Keep rhesus monkeys separate from other species of monkey, in small groups of not more than two to a cage. Ensure full laboratory safety precautions, protective clothing and protection from bites. Avoid skin contamination with saliva. Thoroughly wash any bites and scratch wounds. Periodically screen to control existing infection in a colony using serology and eliminate reactors.

Animals. Inapplicable.

Treatment
Humans.   Symptomatic therapy.

Animals.   Inapplicable.

Vaccination
Humans.   Formalinized   vaccine   has   been   used experimentally.

Animals.   Not applicable.

Legislation
Humans.   The condition is notifiable as acute encephalitis in many countries including the UK, the USA and New Zealand.

Animals.   None.

Histoplasmosis

[Darling's disease, American histoplasmosis]

A dust-borne respiratory infection caused by a dimorphic fungus, in which the parasite phase is yeast-like and the non-parasitic phase in the soil produces a fungal mycelium. It occurs worldwide, but soil of some regions is specially favourable to supporting the fungus.

The causative agent is *Histoplasma capsulatum* (fungus). There is no vaccine.

Reservoir and mode of transmission
Transmitted by inhalation or ingestion of spores in dust from soil contaminated by faeces of birds and bats. Outbreaks have occurred following disturbance of soil and dust by building demolition.

Incubation period
Humans.   5–18 days for primary infection, 3–7 days for reinfection.

Animals.   Unknown.

Clinical features

Humans. Primary pulmonary disease causes influenza-like symptoms with cough, headache and muscle pains. With heavy infection there may be dyspnoea, chest pain, and pericarditis. Erythema nodosum and erythema multiforme may develop. Reinfection may cause miliary lesions in the lungs. Chronic pulmonary infection may occur in people with pre-existing lung disease causing fever, cough, sputum, haemoptysis and cavity formation over months. Disseminated infection may rarely follow primary pulmonary disease and usually occurs in the immunosuppressed and in young children. There are enlarged lymph nodes, liver and spleen, weight loss, ulcerations in the mouth, throat and gastrointestinal tract and possibly endocarditis, chronic meningitis and destruction of adrenal glands.

Animals. Fatal disseminated disease may be seen in dogs but is rare in other animals and birds. Chronic emaciation and diarrhoea may occur.

Pathology

Humans. Infiltration of the hilar lymph nodes may lead to nodule formation, caseous necrosis, calcification and fibrosis in the mediastinum. Nodules in the lungs may give speckled calcification or appear as 'coin' lesions mimicking carcinoma.

Animals. There is diffuse invasion of reticulo-endothelial cells, macrophages and epithelioid cells, without formation of granulomata, to give enlarged lymph nodes, liver and spleen. There is nodular thickening or corrugation of the small intestine and nodules form in the lungs. Intracytoplasmic yeast cells.

Special investigation

Humans and animals. A histoplasma skin test reveals past exposure and is not useful in diagnosing acute infection. Chest X-ray demonstrates calcification. Culture fungus from sputum or infected tissues or stain tissues to demonstrate organism. Serological tests include complement fixation, immunodiffusion and latex agglutination tests.

Prognosis
Humans.   It is usually a subclinical or mild self-limiting illness, although chronic disseminated infection progresses to death unless treated, and may recur after treatment.

Animals.   Progressive, fatal illness is rare and usually in dogs.

Prevention
Humans.   Avoid exposure to dust contaminated by bird or bat faeces in endemic areas. In outbreaks decontaminate soil by spraying with 3% formalin.

Animals.   Impracticable.

Treatment
Humans.   Amphotericin B for disseminated or chronic infection.

Animals.   None.

Legislation
Humans.   Not usually notifiable.

Animals.   None.

Hymenolepiasis

A common but mild tapeworm infection, usually occurring in young children. Occurring worldwide in warm climates, it sometimes causes abdominal pains and diarrhoea.

The causative agents are *Hymenolepis nana* (the dwarf tapeworm of humans) and *H. diminuta* (Cestoda). There is no vaccine.

Reservoir and mode of transmission
The animal reservoir of *H. nana* is the house mouse, but humans can be both definitive and intermediate host. Gravid proglottids disintegrate and eggs pass in the faeces and may be ingested by another human. Larvae then develop in the intestinal villi and pass to the lumen of the

gut to become the adult forms. Dogs, cats and their fleas can be infected as well as grain beetles which can serve as intermediate hosts. The main reservoir of *H. diminuta* is rats, but it requires an intermediate arthropod host (especially flour beetles and moths). Human infection follows ingestion if infected insects infest flour contaminated by rat droppings.

Incubation period
Humans. Prepatent period 2–4 weeks.

Animals. Unknown.

Clinical features
Humans. The condition is usually asymptomatic. Heavy infections may lead to abdominal symptoms including anorexia, diarrhoea and pain, and anal itching.

Animals. Mild catarrhal enteritis with diarrhoea occurs if the infection is heavy.

Pathology
Humans. *H. nana* burrows into intestinal mucosa to form a cercocyst.

Animals. Catarrhal enteritis.

Special investigations
Humans and animals. Identify eggs in faeces.

Prognosis
Humans. Usually asymptomatic or only mild illness.

Animals. Usually subclinical in animals.

Prevention
Humans. Control rodents and protect grain and foodstuffs from *H. diminuta*.

Animals. Impracticable.

Treatment
Humans.   Praziquantel, niclosamide.

Animals.   None.

Legislation
Humans.   Not usually notifiable.

Animals.   None.

Influenza

[Swine and equine influenza, fowl plague]

A respiratory infection, occurring worldwide and sometimes spreading in pandemics, resulting from antigenic
changes in animal strains.

The causative agent is influenza type A (Orthomy-
xoviridae).

Reservoir and mode of transmission

Humans, wild and domestic birds, horses and pigs are reservoirs of influenza viruses, which appear to be species
specific. Transmission is by inhalation of droplets produced by coughing and sneezing, especially in crowded,
enclosed spaces. Convalescent carriers act as reservoir hosts
between epidemics. Antigenic shift is probably required
before animal virus becomes epidemic in humans. Sporadic
human infections with swine and avian strains are reported.

Incubation period

Humans and animals.   1–3 days.

Clinical features

Humans.   Typical symptoms include fever, chills, headache, myalgia, malaise, coryza, pharyngitis and cough with
full recovery within two weeks, although viral or secondary
bacterial pneumonia may develop, especially in the elderly.

Animals.   Fever has a sudden onset followed by anorexia,
coughing, respiratory distress and mucoid nasal discharge,
with rapid recovery.

Pathology
Humans. Interstitial pneumonia, bronchitis and broncho-pneumonia are secondary complications.

Animals. There is consolidation in the lung. Copious mucopurulent exudate fills the bronchioles.

Special investigations
Humans. Isolate virus from nasal and pharyngeal secretions during the acute stage. Serological tests include the haemagglutination inhibition test.

Animals. Serology and virus isolation by chick embryo inoculation.

Prognosis
Humans. There is a high fatality rate during epidemics amongst the elderly and debilitated.

Animals. Mortality is normally low except for poultry affected by fowl plague and foals by equine influenza.

Prevention
Humans. Actively immunize persons at high risk. Amantidine chemoprophylaxis may be indicated in some circumstances.

Animals. Vaccinate horses annually. Prohibit imports of live poultry and poultry meat from countries where fowl plague occurs.

Treatment
Humans. Amantidine.

Animals. None.

Vaccination
Humans. Inactivated vaccines containing prevalent antigens are recommended for persons at special risk of severe disease.

Animals.   Inactivated vaccines are available for horses and pigs.

Legislation
Humans.   None.

Animals.   Fowl plague is notifiable in many countries, with a slaughter policy in the USA, Japan, the UK and some other European countries.

Japanese B encephalitis

[Russian autumnal encephalitis, summer encephalitis, Japanese encephalitis]

A viral encephalitis which may occur in epidemics. It is spread by mosquitoes and has a peak incidence in summer. It is widespread in eastern Asia from Korea to Indonesia, China, India and the western Pacific Islands.

The causative agent is Japanese encephalitis virus (Togaviridae).

Reservoir and mode of transmission
The natural reservoir is probably wild birds, although most horses, pigs and cattle in enzootic areas have antibodies. Pigs, horses and humans are accidental hosts and the titre of virus in the blood is too low to be a source of infection for mosquitoes. Transmission is by mosquito bite. The virus poses a serious hazard to laboratory workers.

Incubation period
Humans.   4–15 days.

Animals.   Unknown.

Clinical features
Humans.   There is acute onset of high fever, with head-ache and prostration, which leads within a few days to encephalitis possibly with spastic paralysis, convulsions and coma.

Animals.   Abortion and neonatal mortality in pigs are features. Signs of encephalitis are seen only occasionally.

Pathology
Humans and animals. A neutrophil leucocytosis occurs. Encephalitis shows perivascular cuffing with neuronal degeneration.

Special investigations
Humans. Isolate virus from the blood and brain. Serological tests include ELISA, haemagglutination inhibition, complement fixation and neutralization tests.

Animals. As for humans, but rarely carried out.

Prognosis
Humans. The fatality rate is 20–50 per cent in encephalitis cases. Permanent neurological damage is common in survivors.

Animals. The neonatal mortality reaches 50–70 per cent. Adults show no clinical signs.

Prevention
Humans. Prevent mosquito bites. Apply strict laboratory safety procedures.

Animals. Vaccinate pigs and horses.

Treatment
Humans. Symptomatic therapy.

Animals. None.

Vaccination
Humans. Mouse brain inactivated virus is offered for children in Japan and some other countries.

Animals. Inactivated tissue culture vaccine is available for pigs and horses.

Legislation
Humans. Acute encephalitis is notifiable in many countries, including the UK and the USA.

Animals. Notifiable in horses in Mexico and some Central and South American countries, Russia and East Germany. There is a slaughter policy in Japan.

Kemerova virus infection

[Tribec virus infections, Kemerova fever]

A tick-borne viral infection of goats and birds that occasionally causes meningo-encephalitis in humans. It occurs worldwide.

The causative agents are the Kemerova viruses (Reoviridae). There is no vaccine.

Reservoir and mode of transmission
The reservoir is a wide range of animals, including goats and birds and their ticks. Transmission is by tick bites.

Incubation period
Humans.   Uncertain, probably 4–5 days.

Animals.   Unknown.

Clinical features
Humans.   There is fever, headache, neck stiffness and possibly neurological signs for a few days.

Animals.   Probably subclinical.

Pathology
Humans.   Meningo-encephalitis.

Animals.   Unknown.

Special investigations
Humans.   Isolate virus from blood or cerebrospinal fluid. Serological tests include the neutralization test.

Animals.   Not done.

Prognosis
Humans.   Usually asymptomatic.

Animals.   Subclinical.

Prevention
Humans.   Avoid tick bites.

Animals.   None.

Treatment
Humans.   Symptomatic therapy.

Animals.   None.

Legislation
Humans.   Acute encephalitis is notifiable in many countries, including the UK and the USA.

Animals.   None.

Kyasanur forest disease

A severe, tick-borne, viral disease which may occur in epidemics. The virus is widespread in India but human infections only occur in villages near the Kyasanur forest of Mysore.

The causative agent is the Kyasanur forest virus (Togaviridae).

Reservoir and mode of transmission

The reservoir is haemaphysal ticks, especially *H. spinigera*, and small mammals, probably rodents and monkeys. Transmission is by tick bites, especially nymphal stages. Ticks remain infective for life and transovarial transmission occurs. Young men working in the forest in the dry season from January to June are principally at risk. Laboratory infections are common.

Incubation period

Humans.   3–8 days.

Animals.   Not known, but probably as for humans.

Clinical features
Humans.   There is sudden onset of fever which may be biphasic, with headache, generalized pains, prostration, conjunctivitis, diarrhoea and vomiting. Vesicles occur on the soft palate. Haemorrhagic manifestations may follow.

Animals.   Deaths have only been observed in monkeys.

Pathology
Humans.   Leucopenia, thrombocytopenia and hae-morrhages.

Animals.   Unknown.

Special investigations
Humans.   Isolate virus from the blood by inoculation into suckling mice or tissue culture. Serological tests include complement fixation, neutralization and haemagglutination tests.

Animals.   None.

Prognosis
Humans.   The fatality rate is 1–10 per cent with prolonged convalescence in survivors.

Animals.   Human infections are preceded by deaths in forest-dwelling Langur and Macacus monkeys. Inapparent infections also occur.

Prevention
Humans.   Avoid tick bites.

Animals.   Control the tick vector.

Treatment
Humans.   Symptomatic therapy.

Animals.   Inappropriate.

Vaccination
Humans.   Experimental only.

Animals. None.

Legislation
Humans and animals. None.

Lassa fever

A severe and often fatal viral haemorrhagic fever spread from wild rodents by contact with their urine. It occurs in western and central Africa, particularly Nigeria, Liberia and Sierra Leone.

The causative agent is the Lassa virus (Arenaviridae). There is no vaccine.

Reservoir and mode of transmission
Reservoirs are wild rodents, especially multimammate rats (*Mastomys natalensis*), which are widely distributed in Africa south of the Sahara. They are infected at birth and remain so for life. Transmission from rodents to humans is by direct or indirect contact with rodent urine on food or in dust, especially during the rainy season when rodents seek shelter indoors. Person-to-person transmission occurs by contact with body fluids, especially through abraded skin, and by aerosol exposure. Laboratory specimens are hazardous.

Incubation period
Humans. 3–17 days, but can be three weeks.

Animals. Unknown.

Clinical features
Humans. Fever has insidious onset over 2–3 days and may persist for up to four weeks, with malaise, headache and generalized aching and sore throat. Vomiting and diarrhoea, possibly oedema of face and neck, lymphadenopathy with haemorrhages and renal failure occurs in the second week. The prostration is out of proportion to fever. Often there is a maculopapular rash.

Animals. Unknown, but probably subclinical.

Pathology
Humans.   Leucopenia and exudative pharyngitis are seen. Later there are petechial haemorrhages, interstitial pneumonitis and fatty degeneration of the liver. An unusual eosinophilic necrosis occurs in the malpighian bodies of the spleen with splenomegaly, and there is focal necrosis in all tissues.

Animals.   Unknown.

Special investigations
Humans.   Isolate the virus from the blood, urine or throat washings. Serological tests include complement fixation and fluorescent antibody tests.

Animals.   Isolate the virus in tissue culture (there appears to be no immune response in the rodent host).

Prognosis
Humans.   The fatality rate is 3–5 per cent with slow recovery of survivors, sometimes leaving persistent deafness.

Animals.   A benign infection in rodents.

Prevention
Humans.   Control rodents. Isolate and barrier-nurse patients. Give medical surveillance to contacts and disinfect all materials and equipment used in nursing. Maximum containment laboratory facilities are required for handling virus.

Animals.   None.

Treatment
Humans.   Symptomatic therapy. Convalescent sera may be used.

Animals.   Inappropriate.

Legislation
Humans.   The disease is notifiable in several countries including the UK, Australia and New Zealand.

Animals.   None.

Leishmaniasis

[*Cutaneous leishmaniasis*: Chiclero ulcer, espundia, pian-bols, uta, and buba (in the Americas); oriental sore, Aleppo boil (in the Old World); Baghdad boil, Delhi boil, Bauru ulcer (in the Middle East).
Visceral leishmaniasis: kala-azar]

A protozoal disease, usually transmitted by flies, which may take the form of a skin ulcer or widespread lesions in the viscera.

The causative agents of cutaneous leishmaniasis are *Leishmania mexicana* and *L. brasiliensis* in the Americas, and *L. tropica* in the Old World; and of visceral leishmaniasis, *L. donovani, L. infantum* and *L. chagasi*. There is no vaccine.

The geographic distribution of the cutaneous disease is Texas, Mexico, Central and South America, India, Pakistan, the Middle East, southern Russia, the Mediterranean coast and Africa. The distribution of visceral leishmaniasis is poorly reported, but foci probably occur in the Mediterranean basin, the Middle East, India, China, Mexico, Central and South America, and Africa.

Reservoir and mode of transmission

Wild animals, dogs and humans serve as reservoirs. Domestic dogs may be an important reservoir for humans. Humans are the only known reservoir in India, infected by the bites of sandfly vectors including *Phlebotomus sergenti* and *P. papatasii*. Person-to-person, congenital and blood-borne transmission of visceral leishmaniasis are possible.

Incubation period

Humans. Cutaneous: one week to several months; visceral: one week to several years.

Animals. For the visceral form in dogs, one month to several years is reported.

Clinical features
Humans.   In the cutaneous disease, the primary lesion is a painful ulcer or nodule at the site of infection persisting for several months, with residual scarring. Further lesions may develop in skin and mucous membranes. In the visceral disease, intermittent irregular fever occurs with sweats, enlarged spleen, weight loss and anaemia leading to ascites, oedema, diarrhoea and secondary infections. Dark pigmentation of the skin may occur.

Animals.   *L. mexicana* causes ulcers of the skin in rodents and other wild animals, usually at the base of the tail. *L. braziliensis* causes a systemic infection with few skin lesions in wild animals. No skin lesions have been found in dogs. Dogs infected by *L. tropica* may suffer from cutaneous lesions similar to those found in humans. *L. donovani* produces visceral lesions in dogs, with enlarged lymph nodes, liver and spleen.

Pathology
Humans.   Infiltration by inflammatory cells at the inoculation site supports the growth of the parasite. This progesses into a large area of chronically inflamed granulation tissue. The overlying skin undergoes hyperplasia and then necrosis with spreading ulceration. Metastatic lesions occur with a similar inflammatory reaction. The lesions may heal, become fibrosed or extend indefinitely to produce considerable disfigurement. In visceral leishmaniasis there is gross enlargement of liver and spleen, and anaemia.

Animals.   In dogs, as for humans. Rodents show only a small ulcer on the skin.

Special investigations
Humans.   Identify organisms in scrapings from lesions. Culture organism from biopsies. An intradermal skin test becomes positive early in illness. Serological tests include ELISA and fluorescent antibody tests.

Animals.   Demonstrate the parasite in lesions or viscera by stained smear and by culture on suitable media; serology.

Prognosis
Humans.   The cutaneous variety ranges from a mild self-limiting infection to a chronic and potentially dangerous metastatic form. *L. braziliensis* is more likely to give rise to chronic infection and disfigurement. The visceral form is usually fatal if untreated but responds well to treatment. Secondary infections (e.g. dysentery) are common.

Animals.   There is an inapparent or chronic skin infection in dogs. The visceral form can be fatal.

Prevention
Humans.   Identify cases and treat. Use insecticides in houses and buildings to control the vector. Avoid sandfly bites. Remove infected dogs.

Animals.   Apply insecticides with a residual action in and around buildings and to vector breeding places. Eliminate rubbish tips and other vector breeding places. Keep dogs indoors after sundown. Remove dog reservoirs.

Treatment
Humans.   Use sodium antimony gluconate and other pentavalent antimonials, and amphotericin B.

Animals.   Not recommended because of the danger of spreading infection.

Legislation
Humans.   Notifiable in a few countries, including Israel, Spain and Italy.

Animals.   Leishmaniasis is notifiable in dogs in Morocco, Cuba and Israel. There is a slaughter policy for affected dogs in Brazil, Spain and Greece.

Leptospirosis

[Weil's disease, haemorrhagic jaundice (*Leptospira icterohaemorrhagiae*), canicola fever (*L. canicola*), dairy worker fever (*L. hardjo*)].

A sporadic bacterial disease of varying severity transmitted by contact with infected animal urine. It occurs worldwide, with areas in which host-adapted serotypes predominate (e.g. *L. hardjo* in cattle in New Zealand and the UK).

The causative agents are Leptospira with over 170 serotypes (bacteria).

Reservoir and mode of transmission

Most animal species may be hosts of leptospires, but the main natural reservoirs for human infection vary with serotype: *L. canicola* in dogs, *L. hardjo* in cattle and *L. icterohaemorrhagiae* in rats. Leptospires are excreted in urine which contaminates the environment, especially water-courses. Humans are infected by direct contact with the animal or contaminated environment and leptospires enter the body through abrasions, wounds or mucous membranes. Person-to-person spread does not occur.

Incubation period

Humans.   3–20 days.

Animals.   1–2 weeks.

Clinical features

Humans.   A wide range of symptoms may accompany fever, including vomiting, headache, muscular pains, conjunctivitis, jaundice, haemolytic anaemia, meningitis, pneumonia and nephritis. Weil's disease is characterized by jaundice and renal failure developing after a few days. *L. hardjo* usually causes an influenza-like illness lasting several days.

Animals.   In cattle, fever and anorexia occur with rapid decline in milk yield and atypical mastitis. Pregnant cows abort with retention of the placenta. In pigs subclinical infection is common, though it can cause abortion and birth of weak piglets. In dogs and cats gastroenteritis, jaundice and nephritis may occur.

Pathology

Humans.   Hepatomegaly with liver degeneration and nephritis occur. Special staining of tissue sections may reveal leptospires.

Animals. Severe acute leptospirosis in ruminants causes mild jaundice and severe anaemia; the liver is enlarged and friable and the kidneys swollen. There may be haemorrhages on serous surfaces. In dogs, *L. icterohaemorrhagiae* produces a marked tendency to haemorrhage, whilst *L. canicola* usually results in chronic interstitial nephritis. Leptospirosis is rare in horses, and in pigs usually results in abortion.

Special investigations
Humans and animals. Serological tests include the microscopic agglutination and complement fixation tests. Isolate the organism from urine by culture or animal (guinea pig or hamster) inoculation (a transport medium is needed to keep the delicate organism alive in transit). Dark-ground microscopy demonstrates motility. Fluorescent antibody staining of urine or culture rapidly demonstrates and identifies certain serotypes.

Prognosis
Humans. Complete recovery is usual, but the fatality rate from Weil's disease may reach 20 per cent.

Animals. *L. canicola* causes chronic nephritis in dogs and eventual death through kidney failure. Considerable loss of production with slow recovery occurs in cattle.

Prevention
Humans. Drain wet ground, control rodents, avoid swimming in or drinking from contaminated waters. Protective clothing is needed for workers at special risk. Impose strict safety rules in laboratories. Immunization in some occupational groups has been advocated. Doxycycline chemoprophylaxis for persons at high exposure for limited periods may be indicated.

Animals. Serologically test before importation. Vaccination a possibility on a herd basis.

Treatment
Humans. Broad-spectrum antibiotics are effective,

especially penicillin and streptomycin. Supportive therapy may be indicated, including renal dialysis.

Animals.   Streptomycin by intramuscular injection during the bacteraemic phase.

Vaccination
Humans.   Killed and attenuated live vaccines are available for some serovars.

Animals.   Available for dogs (*L. canicola* and *L. icterohaemorrhagiae*) and for cattle (*L. hardjo*) repeated annually.

Legislation
Humans.   The disease is notifiable in many countries, including the UK, the USA, Australia and New Zealand. It is a recognized industrial disease in some countries.

Animals.   Laws mainly aim at controlling international trade in live animals. Certain countries insist on negative serological tests before allowing importation. The disease is notifiable in cattle and pigs in many European and Central and South American countries.

Listeriosis

[Mononucleosis, listerellosis, circling disease]

A relatively uncommon, but increasingly recognized, disease in humans worldwide. It occurs mainly in pregnancy, and in neonates, immunosuppressed patients and the elderly. It can cause fatal meningoencephalitis and abortion.

The causative agent is *Listeria monocytogenes* (bacterium). There is no vaccine.

Reservoir and mode of transmission
The agent is widely distributed in animals, birds, humans and soil. The main reservoir for human infection is not clear. The organism is excreted in animal faeces. Outbreaks of food and milk-borne infection have occurred in humans.

Cheese has been identified as a high-risk food. Refriger-
ation of foods may encourage selective growth of listeria.
Cross-infection in hospitals has been reported. Silage used
for fodder may contain heavy infection.

Incubation period
Humans.   Uncertain, but probably a few days.

Animals.   Variable.

Clinical features
Humans.   Symptomless faecal carriage is common. Illness
starts with sudden onset of fever, headache, nausea and
vomiting, and may be followed by meningitis, pneumonia,
septicaemia, endocarditis and localized abscesses. In pregnancy abortion, stillbirth or premature labour may occur
and the infection crosses the placenta to produce neonatal
pneumonia.

Animals.   Two forms exist, the meningoencephalitic and
visceral. The former involves neurological signs with dull-
ness and somnolence. Drooling of saliva and lack of interest in food and mastication soon follow. There is lateral
deviation of the head with a tendency to circle. Paralysis
then sets in with recumbancy and death from respiratory
failure. The visceral form involves abortion, with retained
placenta.

Pathology
Humans.   Granulomatous lesions and abscesses occur in
the liver and other organs and beneath the skin. Focal
necrosis in the placenta with mononuclear infiltration is
seen.

Animals.   Microabscesses occur throughout the brain.
Visceral lesions involve multiple foci of necrosis in the liver,
spleen and heart. Placental lesions are characteristic with
yellow necrotic foci and multiple granulomas in the fetal
liver. Abscess formation in the eye can lead to blindness.

Special investigations
Humans.   Isolate the organism from blood, cerebrospinal

fluid, placenta and amniotic fluid. Storing infected tissues at 4°C allows listeria to grow in preference to most other organisms.

Animals.   Isolate the organism from faeces, urine, milk, aborted fetuses or brain by culture or inoculation into chick embryos or mice.

Prognosis
Humans.   Fatality rates may exceed 20 per cent.

Animals.   Fatality is very high, approaching 3–30 per cent in outbreaks.

Prevention
Humans.   Ensure good personal hygiene and care in the storage and preparation of food. Control cross-infection in hospitalized patients. Heat-treat dairy products. Ensure safe handling of infected animals, and avoid contact with possibly infected materials during pregnancy.

Animals.   Avoid using infected silage, and limit the spread of infection at lambing.

Treatment
Humans.   Various antibiotics such as tetracyclines, chloramphenicol, ampicillin and gentamycin are used.

Animals.   Daily injections of chlortetracycline intra-venously for five days or penicillin intramuscularly for at least seven days in meningoencephalitis cases; this may be followed by relapse.

Legislation
Humans.   Acute meningitis is notifiable in many countries, including the UK, Canada and New Zealand.

Animals.   Notifiable in Peru, Nicaragua, Cuba and some European countries.

Louping Ill

[Ovine encephalomyelitis]

A febrile disease transmitted by ticks. Natural cases are rare in humans and most infections occur in laboratory and slaughterhouse workers, in Scotland, northern England and Wales.

The causative agent is the louping ill virus (Flaviviridae).

Reservoir and mode of transmission

The natural reservoir is sheep, deer, ground-living birds and their ticks (*Ixodes ricinus*). Transmission is by tick bite in spring and early summer when ticks are active. The virus is transmitted from stage to stage but not transovarially in the tick. Transmission to man is by tick bite and possibly aerosol inhalation and accidental inoculation.

Incubation period

Humans.   4–7 days.

Animals.   A few days but sometimes several weeks.

Clinical features

Humans.   Initially there is a fever and influenza-like symptoms, with conjuctivitis, lymphadenitis for 1–2 weeks, followed by an asymptomatic period of a few days and then possibly a return of fever with severe headache, meningism and neurological signs.

Animals.   The infection usually produces mild fever, but when it invades the nervous system it produces signs of encephalitis characterized by incoordination, high-stepping gait, tremors, ataxia and terminal paralysis.

Pathology

Humans.   Uncertain.

Animals.   There is encephalitis with perivascular cuffing typical of non-suppurative encephalomyelitis.

Special investigations
Humans.   Isolate virus from blood and CSF; serology.

Animals.   Isolate virus in chick embryo or tissue culture.

Prognosis
Humans.   No fatalities have been reported, although convalescence may be prolonged.

Animals.   Mortality in enzootic areas is low, but about half the sheep that develop encephalomyelitis die.

Prevention
Humans.   Avoid tick bites and inoculation accidents. Ensure safety in the laboratory.

Animals.   Control ticks by frequent dipping of sheep.

Treatment
Humans.   Symptomatic therapy.

Animals.   None.

Vaccination
Humans.   None.

Animals.   Killed vaccine grown in tissue culture is available. Ewes should be vaccinated in late pregnancy to provide colostral immunity for their lambs.

Legislation
Humans and animals.   None.

Lyme disease

[Lyme arthritis, Bannworth's syndrome, tick-borne meningopolyneuritis, erythema chronicum migrans (ECM), Steere's disease]

A newly recognized, bacterial, tick-borne infection which causes erythema of the skin and in some cases neurological, cardiac and joint disease. The natural reservoir is uncertain. It is enzootic and spreading rapidly in the USA in the coastal areas of the north east, Minnesota, Wisconsin, parts of California and western Nevada; and in Scandinavia and western Europe including Great Britain.

The causative agent is *Borrelia burgdorferi* (bacteria). There is no vaccine.

Reservoir and mode of transmission

The natural reservoirs are believed to be wild rodents, deer and their ticks, *Ixodes ricinus* in Europe, *I. dammini* in eastern USA, and *I. pacificus* in western USA. Human infection is acquired from tick bites, although many cases may not remember being bitten. Dogs also suffer from the disease.

Incubation period

Humans.   Three days to several weeks.

Animals.   Variable.

Clinical features

Humans.   A characteristic erythematous ring, erythema chronicum migrans, occurs at the site of the tick bite; this increases in diameter over days or weeks, with central clearing. There may be multiple lesions with fever and lymphadenopathy, myalgia, headache, abdominal pain and vomiting. Signs of systemic disease may follow weeks to months later: joint pains and arthritis, cardiac arrhythmias and cardiomegaly, and neurological symptoms due to chronic meningitis, cranial nerve palsy or radiculitis.

Animals.   Fever and arthritis are the predominant signs in affected dogs.

Pathology

Humans.   In severe cases, the main lesions include chronic synovitis, erosion of cartilage and bone, pericarditis, meningitis and encephalitis.

Animals.   The infection may cause chronic arthritis in dogs.

Special investigations

Humans. Isolate the organism from skin lesions, blood, cerebrospinal fluid and joint fluid. Serological tests are unsatisfactory at present but include ELISA and indirect immunofluorescence tests: cross-reactions with syphilis are likely.

Animals. Isolate the organism from tissues at post mortem examination. Serology.

Prognosis

Humans. In Europe, systemic illness associated with ECM has been reported infrequently; systemic illness is more common in the USA. Untreated ECM may persist for months. Untreated arthritis may lead to joint destruction.

Animals. It is probably an inapparent infection in free-living mammals, but it causes chronic arthritis in dogs.

Prevention

Humans. Avoid tick-infested areas and tick bites. Early antibiotic treatment of ECM prevents systemic illness.

Animals. Insufficient knowledge.

Treatment

Humans. Tetracyclines and penicillin are used.

Animals. Tetracycline or ampicillin have been used successfully in dogs; otherwise none.

Legislation

Humans. Possibly notifiable as meningitis in some countries.

Animals. None.

Lymphocytic choriomeningitis

[LCM encephalomyelitis, LCM, Armstrong's disease]

A febrile, viral infection occurring worldwide, which may

progress to meningitis. It is transmitted to humans from rodents.

The causative agent is lymphocytic choriomeningitis virus (Arenaviridae). There is no vaccine.

Reservoir and mode of transmission

The reservoir is domestic mice (*Mus musculus*). Infection is maintained in mice by congenital infection followed by life-long carriage and excretion of virus in saliva, urine and faeces. Human infections are probably from contaminated food and dust, the handling of dead mice, and mouse bites. Infections in the laboratory are common. Laboratory and pet hamsters have caused outbreaks in the USA and Germany. Person-to-person spread has not been reported.

Incubation period

Humans.   6–13 days.

Animals.   Variable.

Clinical features

Humans.   The features may include influenza-like illness for up to two weeks, possibly with orchitis. Sometimes meningitis, paralysis and coma follow. Joint pains occur during convalescence.

Animals.   The condition usually remains subclinical in natural infection, but in experimentally infected fetal mice there is stunted growth. Adult mice show convulsions and may die. Survivors show full recovery.

Pathology

Humans.   Lymphocytic meningoencephalitis is characteristic.

Animals.   Glomerular nephritis and meningitis with destruction of neurones occurs after experimental infection.

Special investigations

Humans.   Isolate the virus from blood, nasopharynx or cerebrospinal fluid. Serological tests include the complement fixation and indirect fluorescent antibody tests.

Animals.　Serology; isolate the virus in tissue culture and demonstrate its presence in tissues by immunofluorescence.

Prognosis
Humans.　Fatality is rare.

Animals.　Subclinical infection is usual, but outbreaks with high fatality can occur in laboratory rodents owing to suppression of immunity.

Prevention
Humans.　Control and avoid contact with rodents. Apply strict laboratory safety procedures.

Animals.　Impracticable.

Treatment
Humans.　Symptomatic therapy.

Animals.　None.

Legislation
Humans.　Aseptic or viral meningitis is notifiable in some countries, including the UK, Canada and the USA.

Animals.　None.

Marburg disease

[Green monkey disease]

A rare and often fatal viral haemorrhagic fever of laboratory personnel. The disease originates from East Africa and is spread by monkeys transported for laboratory work.

　　The causative agent is the Marburg virus (Rhabdoviridae). There is no vaccine.

Reservoir and mode of transmission

Cases occur in people in direct contact with organs and fluids of African green (vervet) laboratory monkeys

(*Cercopithecus aethiops*), but extensive studies have not incriminated the green monkey or any other wild mammal as the natural reservoir. Person-to-person transmission by contact with infected blood occurs especially in hospitals and by sexual transmission via semen.

Incubation period
Humans. 3–9 days.

Animals. As for humans in experimental infections.

Clinical features
Humans. Fever, which persists for 10–20 days, has sudden onset with rigors, headache and generalized pains, anorexia, vomiting and diarrhoea; this sometimes leads to dehydration, conjunctivitis, pharyngitis, enanthem on palate, maculopapular rash, jaundice, haemorrhagic manifestations and renal failure. The rash appears between the third and eighth days of illness and lasts for 3–4 days. Death, if it occurs, is usually at the beginning of the second week.

Animals. None known in the wild, though experimentally infected monkeys usually die following fever and anorexia.

Pathology
Humans. Leucopenia, thrombocytopenia, focal necrosis and haemorrhage in all organs are the main changes.

Animals. Leucopenia and petechial haemorrhages throughout the body of experimentally infected monkeys, sometimes with gastrointestinal haemorrhages.

Special investigations
Humans and animals. Isolate virus from blood, urine and pharyngeal secretions; serology.

Prognosis
Humans. The case fatality rate is about 25 per cent.

Animals. No clinical signs occur in green monkeys, but the disease is usually fatal after experimental infection of other primate species.

Prevention
Humans. Strictly isolate patients and place contacts under daily surveillance for 21 days. Avoid inoculation accidents and use maximum laboratory containment facilities when handling the virus.

Animals. Impossible at present owing to lack of knowledge.

Treatment
Humans. Symptomatic and supportive therapy. Specific immunoglobulin may be available.

Animals. None.

Legislation
Humans. The disease is notifiable in the UK, Australia, New Zealand and some European countries.

Animals. None.

Mayaro and sindbis fevers

[Jungle fever]

A benign, febrile, viral disease which can progress to swelling of joints and to jaundice. It is transmitted by mosquitoes to humans entering forest areas.

The causative agents are Mayaro and Sindbis viruses (Togaviridae). There is no vaccine.

The Mayaro virus occurs in South America, principally Trinidad and Brazil; the Sindbis virus occurs in Africa, India, South East Asia, the Philippines, Australia and Europe.

Reservoir and mode of transmission
Virus has been isolated from wild animals, birds and mosquitoes. Transmission is by mosquito bite, humans being an accidental host when entering areas where the virus cycles between wild animals and mosquitoes. Laboratory-acquired infections also occur. Infection of wildfowl has been associated with the Sindbis virus.

Incubation period
Humans. Probably 3–12 days.

Animals. Not known.

Clinical features
Humans. Symptoms of a few days duration include fever, severe headache, generalized pains, rigors, jaundice, a maculopapular rash at onset or within 1–2 days of the start of symptoms, pain and swelling of joints, especially of the feet and hands.

Animals. Unknown.

Pathology
Humans. Uncertain.

Animals. Unknown.

Special investigations
Humans and animals. Isolate virus from blood. Serological tests include haemagglutination inhibition, neutralization and complement fixation tests.

Prognosis
Humans. The condition is usually benign with full recovery, but the joint pains may persist for several weeks.

Animals. No signs recognized.

Prevention
Humans. Control mosquitoes and avoid bites. Ensure laboratory safety.

Animals. Control the mosquito vector.

Treatment
Humans. Symptomatic therapy.

Animals. None.

Legislation

Humans and animals.　None.

Melioidosis

[Pseudo-glanders, Whitmore's disease]

A chronic, febrile, respiratory bacterial disease acquired by direct contact with infected animals and the environment. It occurs in tropical and subtropical regions, especially South East Asia, North East Australia, Central America and the Caribbean areas.

The causative agent is *Pseudomonas pseudomallei* (bacterium). There is no vaccine.

Reservoir and mode of transmission

The main reservoirs are pigs, sheep and goats, and soil and water. Transmission is more frequent in wet conditions by contamination of wounds, abrasions or by inoculation. Pulmonary disease may result from inhalation of dust. Laboratory accidents have occurred.

Incubation period

Humans and animals.　Two days to many years.

Clinical features

Humans.　Highly variable symptoms include: pulmonary disease with cough, sputum, chest pain and fever; septicaemia; osteomyelitis; subcutaneous abscesses.

Animals.　Signs include loss of weight, swelling of joints, fever, coughing and dyspnoea. Sheep become recumbent and some die.

Pathology

Humans and animals.　Initial septicaemia is followed by localization of infection in various organs, producing multiple abscesses in lungs, liver and spleen. Joint infection leads to polyarthritis with large quantities of pus. Ulcers may occur.

Special investigations

Humans.　Isolate the organism from sputum, urine, pus and blood. Serological tests include complement fixation, haemagglutination and agglutination tests.

Animals. Isolate the organism from nasal discharge or pus; use guinea pig or rabbit inoculation; serology; allergic skin test using melioidin as antigen.

Prognosis
Humans. Subclinical infection appears to be common. The infection may be latent, causing symptoms many years after exposure. Disseminated disease is more common in debilitated patients.

Animals. Sheep seem especially susceptible. The joint lesions become fibrosed with persistent induration. Over 25 per cent mortality can occur in outbreaks.

Prevention
Humans. Avoid contamination of wounds. Apply strict laboratory procedures.

Animals. Prohibit or quarantine imports of animals from infected countries. Control rodents and destroy infected domestic animals. Cleanse and disinfect contaminated premises and equipment.

Treatment
Humans. Broad-spectrum antibiotics.

Animals. Unlikely to be undertaken. Supportive therapy with antibiotics is sometimes tried.

Legislation
Humans. None.

Animals. Notifiable in Argentina, some Central American countries and Caribbean islands, Korea, Malaysia and New Zealand.

Monkeypox

A rare and sporadic viral disease, usually of children, transmitted from monkeys and resembling smallpox. It was only recognized after the eradication of smallpox, and occurs in

the tropical rain forests of central and western Africa.
    The causative agent is the monkeypox virus (Poxviridae).

Reservoir and mode of transmission
Outbreaks have occurred in captive Asiatic monkeys. The
virus has been isolated from a wild squirrel. Transmission
to humans probably occurs by inhalation or direct contact
with virus excreted by monkeys, squirrels or from carcasses. Secondary person-to-person spread does occur but
less frequently than for smallpox. The virus poses a major
hazard to laboratory workers.

Incubation period
Humans.   7–17 days.

Animals.   Probably as for humans.

Clinical features
Humans.   The illness of 2–4 weeks duration begins usually
with fever, severe headache, backache, malaise, prostration and generalized lymphadenopathy, and is followed 1–3
days later by a generalized rash particularly prominent on
the face, palms and feet. Skin lesions progress from
macules to papules, pustules and scabs. Sore throat and
cough may be reported and severe complications include
bronchopneumonia, vomiting and diarrhoea.

Animals.   There are multiple, raised, widely distributed
lesions.

Pathology
Humans and animals.   Skin and mucous membrane
lesions consist of vesicular pocks which umbilicate, scab
and fall off. Secondary bacterial infection may occur.

Special investigations
Humans.   Isolate virus from skin lesions. Serological tests
include haemagglutination inhibition, fluorescent antibody, ELISA and radioimmunoassay tests.

Animals.   Isolate virus in tissue culture or in
embryonating eggs. Haemorrhagic ulcers form on the

chicken chorio-allantoic membrane. Infected cells show brick-shaped intracytoplasmic inclusion bodies on staining.

Prognosis
Humans. The case fatality rate in unvaccinated subjects is up to 16 per cent.

Animals. Fatality is rare. The skin lesions can be few and benign but wide dissemination occurs.

Prevention
Humans. Strictly isolate patients and monitor contacts. Apply strict laboratory safety procedures. Vaccinate laboratory staff.

Animals. Impossible at present owing to lack of knowledge.

Treatment
Humans. Symptomatic therapy.

Animals. None.

Vaccination
Humans. Smallpox vaccination protects and should be offered to laboratory workers who handle the virus.

Animals. None.

Legislation
Humans and animals. None.

Mucambo fever

A mild, febrile, viral disease in South America and the West Indies.

The causative agent is the mucambo virus (Togaviridae). There is no vaccine.

Reservoir and mode of transmission
The disease is endemic in wild rodents and other animals, including mosquitoes, and is maintained by a mosquito vector. Transmission to humans is presumably via mosquito bites.

Incubation period
Humans.   Uncertain.

Animals.   Unknown.

Clinical features
Humans.   Features include mild fever, headache and generalized pains for a few days.

Animals.   Unknown.

Pathology
Humans and animals.   Unknown.

Special investigations
Humans.   Isolate virus from blood. Serological tests include haemagglutination inhibition, complement fixation and neutralization tests.

Animals.   Not usually applicable.

Prognosis
Humans.   It is a self-limiting and mild illness.

Animals.   Unknown.

Prevention
Humans.   Avoid mosquito bites.

Animals.   None.

Treatment
Humans.   Symptomatic therapy.

Animals.   None.

Legislation
Humans and animals.   None.

Murray Valley encephalitis

[Australian encephalitis]

A severe, sometimes fatal, viral fever and encephalitis, occurring in Australia and New Guinea.

The causative agents are several flaviviruses (Togaviridae). There is no vaccine.

Reservoir and mode of transmission

The virus circulates between birds and mosquitoes. An outbreak of Murray Valley encephalitis in south eastern Australia in the early 1950s followed the southerly migration of water birds because of heavy rainfall in the north where infection is endemic. The virus poses a serious hazard to laboratory workers.

Incubation period

Humans.   Probably 5–15 days.

Animals.   Unknown.

Clinical features

Humans. Fever begins suddenly with headache, anorexia, vomiting, meningism and neurological signs. Recovery or death is usual within two weeks.

Animals.   Subclinical.

Pathology

Humans.   Encephalitis.

Animals.   Unknown.

Special investigations

Humans. Serological tests include haemagglutination inhibition and complement fixation tests. Isolate virus from the brain post mortem.

Animals.   Demonstration of these viruses is difficult.

Prognosis
Humans.   Subclinical infection is common, but case fatality reaches 20–60 per cent in children. Neurological and psychiatric sequelae persist in some survivors.

Animals.   This infection is mainly subclinical.

Prevention
Humans.   Control mosquito vectors and avoid their bites. Apply strict laboratory safety procedures.

Animals.   Not applicable.

Treatment
Humans.   Symptomatic therapy.

Animals.   Not required.

Legislation
Humans.   Acute encephalitis is notifiable in many countries, including the UK and the USA.

Animals.   None.

Mycobacterial infection (opportunist)

[Atypical mycobacteria infection]

An unusual, opportunist, bacterial infection resembling tuberculosis. It occurs usually in immunosuppressed persons, and appears worldwide.

The causative agents are several Mycobacterium species, including *M. avium* and *M. marinum* (bacterium). There is no vaccine.

Reservoir and mode of transmission
Several species of atypical mycobacteria contaminate the environment but do not always have a natural host. They are opportunist infections of humans and animals. *M. marinum* appears to infect fish and may be transmitted to humans from contaminated aquaria, water-courses used

for swimming, and fish or marine mammal bites. The reservoir of *M. avium* is wild and domesticated birds and poultry, and human infection presumably results from inhalation of infected dust or during the preparation of carcasses.

Incubation period
Humans.   Uncertain.

Animals.   Variable.

Clinical features
Humans.   *M. marinum* resulting from wound infection causes abscess formation which may take months to heal. *M. avium* may cause respiratory symptoms resembling tuberculosis with lymphadenitis.

Animals.   Ill-thrift in poultry due to *M. avium*.

Pathology
Humans.   There are granulomata which may not caseate.

Animals.   In birds there are disseminated granulomata in the liver, spleen, intestines and bone marrow. Lesions do not undergo caseation or calcification. In pigs lesions occur in the lymph nodes of the neck.

Special investigations
Humans and animals.   Isolate mycobacteria from sputum or abscesses. Stain sections to reveal acid-fast rods.

Prognosis
Humans.   Atypical mycobacteria usually cause opportunist infections in immunosuppressed or debilitated patients (e.g. AIDS patients), whose prognosis is poor.

Animals.   Wild birds and poultry can show progressive and fatal disease. Cattle and sheep rarely show clinical signs. Some strains of atypical mycobacteria mimic *M. johnei* in housed goats and sheep. Pigs show no signs of infection but infected heads must be condemned.

Prevention
Humans. Drain and clean contaminated swimming pools and aquaria.

Animals. Avoid contact with wild birds.

Treatment
Humans. Tuberculosis chemotherapy is used but may be unsuccessful. Drain abscesses.

Animals. None.

Legislation
Humans. Tuberculosis is a notifiable disease in most countries.

Animals. None.

Newcastle disease

[Newcastle fever, pseudo fowl pest]

A rare cause of viral conjunctivitis. It occurs worldwide and is spread from infected birds to occupationally exposed persons.

The causative agent is Newcastle disease virus (Paramyxoviridae).

Reservoir and mode of transmission
The natural reservoir is wild and domesticated birds. Transmission is by inhalation of infectious aerosols. Intensive conditions favour spread by contact, on inanimate objects and air-borne between poultry houses. Human infections occur mainly amongst laboratory workers and those who work with infected chickens or who give live vaccine, especially by aerosol.

Incubation period
Humans. 1–2 days.

Animals. 5–6 days.

Clinical features
Humans. Usually symptoms are confined to painful conjunctivitis lasting a few days, but fever and influenza-like symptoms for up to three weeks may follow.

Animals. In poultry, respiratory and nervous signs occur, including gasping and coughing; also drooping of wings, twisting of the head and neck; inappetence and paralysis. Egg production ceases.

Pathology
Humans. Non-specific lesions of acute inflammation occur.

Animals. Petechial haemorrhages are characteristic, especially in the proventricular mucosa. Necrosis of the intestinal mucosa gives a 'bran' like appearance. Congestion and mucoid exudate appears in the lungs and bronchi.

Special investigations
Humans. Isolate virus from eye washings, blood and urine. Serological tests include the neutralization test.

Animals. Isolate virus in chick embryos or tissue culture. An agglutination test using red blood cells of various animal species can be used. Strains are graded by virulence into velogenic–viscerotropic, velogenic–neurotropic, mesogenic and lentogenic types. Virulence is determined by three tests: mean death time of chick embryos, intracerebral pathogenicity in day-old chicks, and intravenous pathogenicity in six-week-old chickens. Serology is also used.

Prognosis
Humans. It is a mild self-limiting infection.

Animals. Mortality is 90 per cent or more from velogenic–viscerotropic and 10–15 per cent in velogenic-neurotropic disease; the mesotropic form is less severe and the lentogenic is mild or inapparent. The virus can also cause meningoencephalitis and death in mink.

Prevention
Humans.   Hygienic precautions are needed when handling infected birds. Avoid inoculation injuries and ensure laboratory safety.

Animals.   Maintain strict hygiene in poultry sheds, physical separation of poultry houses, quarantine of imported live birds, prohibition of imports from infected countries, sterilization of, or prohibition on, waste food fed to poultry. Vaccination is commonly practised.

Treatment
Humans.   Symptomatic therapy.

Animals.   None.

Vaccination
Humans.   None.

Animals.   Inactivated or live vaccines of varying virulence may be used depending on the likely challenge. Lentogenic strains of vaccine are usually given in drinking water, by intranasal or intraocular instillation, by dusting or by aerosol fogging. Mesogenic and inactivated vaccines must be given individually. Choice of vaccine is subject to state control in the UK.

Legislation
Humans.   None.

Animals.   The disease is notifiable in most parts of the world. A slaughter policy is only adopted when the disease incidence has been reduced to a low level by vaccination and other control measures.

Omsk haemorrhagic fever

A severe viral haemorrhagic fever affecting rural workers and their children in wet grassland and swamp areas near Omsk and Novosibirsk in western Siberia. It is transmitted by ticks from rodents.

The causative agent is the Omsk haemorrhagic fever virus (Togaviridae).

Reservoir and mode of transmission

The natural reservoir is rodents, muskrats and possibly ticks. Transmission is by the bite of infective ticks (possibly *Dermacentor pictus* and *D. marginatus*) and by direct contact with muskrats which were introduced for hunting in the 1920s. A cycle involving ticks and rodents exists but is not fully understood.

Incubation period

Humans.   3–8 days.

Animals.   Unknown.

Clinical features

Humans.   There is sudden onset of fever which may be biphasic, with headache, generalized pains, prostration, conjunctivitis, diarrhoea and vomiting. Vesicles occur on the soft palate. Haemorrhagic manifestations may follow.

Animals.   Deaths are only observed in monkeys.

Pathology

Humans.   Leucopenia, thrombocytopenia and haemorrhages.

Animals.   Unknown.

Special investigations

Humans.   Isolate virus from the blood in suckling mice, and in tissue culture. Serological tests include complement fixation, neutralization and haemagglutination tests.

Animals.   Not usually undertaken.

Prognosis

Humans.   The fatality rate is 1–10 per cent.

Animals.   Inapparent infections occur.

Prevention
Humans.   Avoid areas of tick activity and tick bites.

Animals.   Control the tick vector.

Treatment
Humans.   Symptomatic therapy.

Animals.   Inappropriate.

Vaccination
Humans.   Experimental only.

Animals.   None.

Legislation
Humans.   Cases imported to the UK would be notifiable as viral haemorrhagic fever.

Animals.   None.

Opisthorchiasis

A relatively mild liver fluke infection acquired by eating raw fish. It occurs in the USSR, southern and central Europe, India, the Far East and the Americas.

The causative agents are *Opisthorchis felineus* (*tenuicollis*), *O. oviverrini, O. pseudofilineus, O. sinensis* and *Pseudamphistomum truncatum* (Trematoda). There is no vaccine.

Reservoir and mode of transmission
The parasite lodges in the bile ducts of the definitive hosts, which are any animals that eat raw fish including humans, dogs and cats. Eggs in the faeces hatch into miracidiae, which are then eaten by snails and develop into cercariae, which penetrate tissues of freshwater fish, which in turn eat the snails. Cercariae develop into metacercariae, which migrate into the bile ducts of definitive hosts after they eat the fish.

Incubation period
Humans. Variable, up to many years.

Animals. Presumably as for humans.

Clinical features
Humans. The condition is often asymptomatic. Symptoms follow obstruction of bile ducts: anorexia, abdominal discomfort, hepatomegaly, jaundice, cirrhosis.

Animals. It is mild if parasites are few. Heavy infections give liver enlargement.

Pathology
Humans. Obstruction of bile ducts leads to cholangitis, portal cirrhosis, and possibly carcinoma of the liver.

Animals. Chronic cirrhosis with cholangitis occurs in dogs and cats.

Special investigations
Humans and animals. Identify characteristic eggs in faeces.

Prognosis
Humans. This depends on the number of worms present. Light infections may be asymptomatic. Heavy chronic infection leads to cirrhosis and death.

Animals. Light infections are subclinical.

Prevention
Humans. Cooking, prolonged freezing or salt treatment of freshwater fish kill the parasites. Dispose of faeces with sanitary precautions.

Animals. Freeze fish or cook thoroughly before feeding to cats or dogs.

Treatment
Humans. Praziquantel.

Animals.   Oral chloroquine or praziquantel.

Legislation
Humans and animals.   None.

Orf

[Contagious pustular dermatitis, contagious ecthyma of sheep, contagious pustular stomatitis]

A viral skin infection, occurring worldwide, acquired from infected sheep. It appears during spring in people tending lambs and again in autumn in slaughterhouse workers.
   The causative agent is orf virus (Poxviridae).

Reservoir and mode of transmission
The natural reservoirs are sheep and goats. Transmission of virus from superficial lesions is by direct and indirect contact, with entry through skin abrasions. Tough forage, likely to injure the lips, facilitates infection in animals. Lambs and kids transmit infection from their mouth lesions to teats and udders when suckling. Infection may persist from season to season in scabs on pasture or possibly in carrier animals. The virus is highly resistant to adverse environments and persists for many years.

Incubation period
Humans.   3–6 days.

Animals.   2–3 days.

Clinical features
Humans.   Usually there is a single painful red primary lesion on the hand or forearm lasting 3–6 weeks. The lesions progress from a macule to a papule and finally to a pustule. The centre of the pustule sinks and there is weeping of fluid. Secondary bacterial infection may occur.

Animals.   Lesions on the lips, nostrils and ears pass through papular, vesicular and pustular stages finishing after 10–12 days in thick brown scabs. Intense pain can interfere with eating.

Pathology
Humans and animals. Lesions begin as papules progressing to vesicles and pustules which scab and heal.

Special investigations
Humans and animals. Identify the virus by electron microscopy of lesion fluid.

Prognosis
Humans. It is a benign self-limiting infection.

Animals. The fatality rate is low and generally due to secondary infection or fly strike. Loss of condition occurs in severe cases, where painful lesions around the mouth interfere with feeding.

Prevention
Humans. Wash hands after contact with infected animals.

Animals. Vaccinate and avoid rough pasture on farms where the infection is severe.

Treatment
Humans and animals. Antibiotics are given against secondary infection.

Vaccination
Humans. None.

Animals. Live, virulent vaccine is applied by scarification of the skin of the axilla.

Legislation
Humans and animals. None.

Oropouche fever

[Oropouche virus disease]

A relatively benign and self-limiting febrile viral disease which occurs in large epidemics in urban areas of South

America and Trinidad. The disease is endemic in certain forests.

The causative agent is the Oropouche virus (Bunyaviridae). There is no vaccine.

Reservoir and mode of transmission

The natural reservoir is in wild animals, especially monkeys, sloths and birds. Transmission appears to be due to midge and mosquito bites. The virus poses a serious hazard to laboratory workers.

Incubation period

Humans.　Probably about 3–12 days.

Animals.　Unknown.

Clinical features

Humans.　Fever has a sudden onset, with severe headache, generalized joint and muscle pains, chills, dizziness and photophobia lasting up to a week.

Animals.　Unknown, but probably subclinical.

Pathology

Humans.　Leucopenia occurs.

Animals.　Unknown.

Special investigations

Humans.　Isolate virus from blood. Serological tests include haemagglutination inhibition and neutralization tests.

Animals.　None.

Prognosis

Humans.　It is a benign, self-limiting illness.

Animals.　Unknown.

Prevention

Humans.　Insufficient information exists to control urban

epidemics. Avoid midge and mosquito bites. Apply strict laboratory safety procedures.

Animals.   None.

Treatment
Humans.   Symptomatic therapy.

Animals.   None.

Legislation
Humans and animals.   None.

Paragonimiasis

[Pulmonary distomatosis, endemic or oriental hemoptysis, lung fluke disease]

A respiratory fluke infection acquired by consuming uncooked crayfish and crabs. It occurs in South East Asia, especially Korea, Japan, China, Taiwan, the Philippines, West Africa and the Pacific coast of South America.

The causative agents are several species of Paragonimus. *P. westermani* is the most important (Trematode). There is no vaccine.

Reservoir and mode of transmission
Definitive hosts include wild felines, pigs, dogs, cats, monkeys and rodents which are infected on eating raw crab or crayfish. The adult worm encysts in the bronchioles. Eggs are coughed up, swallowed and passed in the faeces. Two intermediate hosts are needed, including a snail and then a freshwater crayfish or crab. Cercariae develop in the snail and then into metacercariae in the crayfish. Metacercariae penetrate the intestines and migrate through the abdominal and thoracic cavities into the lung to complete the life-cycle. Humans are infected by eating uncooked crayfish or food secondarily contaminated with metacercariae from crab or crayfish, or by eating raw meat from wild animals containing migrating larvae.

Incubation period
Humans.   Variable.

Animals. Unknown, but infection reaches the lung in 23–35 days after ingestion.

Clinical features
Humans. Fever has an insidious onset, with chronic cough, red-coloured sputum owing to the large number of eggs, haemoptysis, chest pain, dyspnoea and bronchiectasis. Neurological symptoms (e.g. fits, paraplegia) follow migration of the fluke into the brain and spinal cord. Symptoms may persist for years.

Animals. With heavy infestation coughing occurs with bloody sputum. Signs of bronchitis and bronchopneumonia are seen with weakness and lethargy.

Pathology
Humans. The migrating worms provoke inflammation and abscess formation in the abdominal and thoracic cavities. Cysts form with granulomatous reaction surrounding eggs in the lung tissue. Worms may migrate from lungs to brain and other organs through soft tissues to form cysts. Eggs may be transported to other organs, provoking granulomatous reaction. There is usually a moderate eosinophilia.

Animals. As for humans in dogs and cats.

Special investigations
Humans and animals. X-ray the lungs to show small cavities containing worms. Identify characteristic eggs in faeces and sputum. Serological tests include counterimmunofluorescence and complement fixation tests.

Prognosis
Humans. Chronic infection persists as a bronchopneumonia with bronchiectasis. Extrapulmonary infection, though rare, results in serious damage to the brain.

Animals. Chronic non-fatal disease occurs.

Prevention
Humans.   Avoid eating raw crabs, crayfish and meat. Practise good food hygiene techniques.

Animals.   Dispose of sewage with efficient filtration and processing of effluent. Control snails using molluscicides. Prevent domestic animals from eating raw crayfish and shrimps.

Treatment
Humans.   Praziquantel.

Animals.   Bithional.

Legislation
Humans and animals.   None.

Paravaccinia

[Pseudocowpox, milkers' nodules, bovine papular stomatitis]

A benign viral infection, occurring worldwide, acquired by contact with infected cows.
   The causative agent is paravaccinia virus (Poxviridae). There is no vaccine.

Reservoir and mode of transmission
Pseudocowpox on cows' teats and bovine papular stomatitis in calves' mouths are thought to be caused by the same virus, direct transmission occurring during suckling. Milkers are infected through skin abrasions, and there is mechanical transmission amongst cows on milking equipment.

Incubation period
Humans and animals.   Probably up to one week.

Clinical features
Humans.   Small, painful nodules erupt on the hands and forearms and last for up to six weeks.

Animals.   Papules, progressing to pustules, occur on teats. They tend to recur.

Pathology
Humans and animals. Foci of erythema develop into papules with a central vesicle which becomes pustular, scabs and heals.

Special investigations
Humans and animals. Demonstrate virus particles by electron microscopy of lesion fluid.

Prognosis
Humans. It is a mild self-limiting infection.

Animals. It is a mild epithelial infection. Mastitis is a likely complication in cows. There may be interference with milking owing to painful sores.

Prevention
Humans. Practise good dairy hygiene.

Animals. Practise good dairy hygiene and always milk affected cows last.

Treatment
Humans. None.

Animals. None except topical therapy on teats.

Legislation
Humans and animals. None.

Pasteurellosis

[Shipping or transport fever, haemorrhagic septicaemia]

A common bacterial wound infection resulting from animal bites. It occurs worldwide.

The causative agents are the Pasteurella species, usually *P. multocida* (bacterium).

Reservoir and mode of transmission
All animals and birds may be colonized by pasteurellas, and human infection occurs by wound infection from bites or

scratches. Animal-to-animal transmission may occur by ingestion and inhalation.

Incubation period
Humans. Up to 48 hours from the bite to the onset of inflammatory reaction.

Animals. Variable.

Clinical features
Humans. Local inflammation occurs around the bite or scratch, possibly leading to abscess formation with systemic symptoms.

Animals. Very variable, from mild subclinical involvement to fever, severe respiratory disease and death.

Pathology
Humans. Not specific.

Animals. In haemorrhagic septicaemia there is congestion, oedema, excess fluid (often blood-stained) in serous cavities, petechial haemorrhages and acute congestion of the lungs.

Special investigations
Humans and animals. Isolate the causal agent from the wound or lesion.

Prognosis
Humans. Although the disease is usually self-limiting, septicaemia is possible but rarely fatal.

Animals. Acute and peracute infection in animals can cause fatal pneumonia and septicaemia. Dogs and cats are frequently healthy carriers.

Prevention
Humans and animals. Avoid bites and scratches. Destroy aggressive stray dogs and cats. Attend to hygienic care of wounds.

Treatment
Humans and animals.   Broad-spectrum antibiotics.

Vaccination
Humans.   None.

Animals.   Vaccine is available for cattle and sheep but is not used in companion animals.

Legislation
Humans and animals.   None.

Piry fever

A poorly documented viral fever acquired from mosquito bites. It has occurred in Brazil.

The causative agent is the Piry virus (Rhabdoviridae). There is no vaccine.

Reservoir and mode of transmission
Serological evidence suggests that a wide range of animals, including humans, is infected. The virus has been isolated from the possum and transmission is believed to be by mosquito bite and by laboratory accident.

Incubation period
Humans.   Uncertain, but probably up to one week.

Animals.   Unknown.

Clinical features
Humans.   There is sudden onset of fever, headache, backache, generalized pains, photophobia, and pharyngitis for a few days.

Animals.   Unknown.

Pathology
Humans.   Not specific.

Animals.   Unknown.

Special investigations
Humans. Isolate virus from blood. Serological tests include complement fixation and neutralization tests.

Animals. None.

Prognosis
Humans. It is a benign, self-limiting infection.

Animals. Presumably subclinical.

Prevention
Humans. Avoid mosquito bites.

Animals. None.

Treatment
Humans. Symptomatic therapy.

Animals. None.

Legislation
Humans and animals. None.

Plague

[Pest, black death, pestilential fever]

A highly dangerous bacterial infection. It is transmitted by rat fleas and from person to person, and may occur in large epidemics. Its geographical distribution is western USA, South America and Asia.

The causative agent is *Yersinia pestis* (bacterium).

Reservoir and mode of transmission
The natural source of bubonic plague is the brown rat (*Rattus norvegicus*) and the rat fleas, *Xenopsylla cheopis* and *Ceratophyllus fasciatus*. The flea ingests infected blood, and *Y. pestis* multiplies in the flea's stomach and is excreted in its faeces or is regurgitated. Rats are infected by flea bites. Humans are infected by rat flea bites, or by handling infected rats, or by person-to-person droplet spread (pneumonic plague). The death of infected rats

causes fleas to seek other hosts such as the black rat (*Rattus rattus*) which carry fleas into close contact with humans. Specimens and cultures are hazardous for laboratory workers.

Incubation period
Humans and animals.   2–6 days.

Clinical features
Humans.   Bubonic plague causes painful suppuration of lymph nodes draining the bite, with fever, cough and sometimes neurological signs which may rapidly progress to death within a few days. Haemorrhages and ischaemic necrosis of the skin causes black patches. Pneumonic plague causes fever, cough, pneumonia and septicaemia.

Animals.   Rodents develop clinical signs similar to humans and are often found dead. Carnivores suffer only mild fever.

Pathology
Humans.   There are enlarged, hard, congested, haemorrhagic and necrotic lymph nodes containing bacteria with pus (so-called buboes). Haemorrhages occur throughout the body and there is acute and haemorrhagic pneumonia. Disseminated intravascular coagulation takes place and areas of skin undergo necrosis (hence 'black death').

Animals.   A pustule may develop at the site of the flea bite. Infection spreads in lymphatics to regional lymph nodes which undergo acute inflammation. Bacteraemia follows with suppurative foci throughout the body. Endotoxins induce intravascular clotting, causing widespread multiple embolism and necrosis.

Special investigations
Humans and animals.   Identify the pathogens by microscopy of sputum or pus. Isolate *Y. pestis* from blood, pus or sputum.

Prognosis
Humans. Bubonic plague has a case fatality rate of over 50 per cent. Pneumonic plague is usually fatal unless treated early.

Animals. Infected rats and squirrels frequently die unless they are from an enzootic area and have acquired immunity.

Prevention
Humans. Isolate and treat all cases. Keep contacts under surveillance or quarantine. Apply rodenticides and insecticides. Immunize travellers to endemic areas. Give chemoprophylaxis to contacts using tetracycline or sulphonamides. Apply strict laboratory safety procedures.

Animals. None.

Treatment
Humans. Streptomycin, tetracyline or chloramphenicol are effective in early illness.

Animals. Inappropriate.

Vaccination
Humans. Inactivated vaccine protects only for six months but is recommended for travellers and tourists in endemic areas, and for laboratory staff.

Animals. Inappropriate.

Legislation
Humans. Notify internationally (WHO). Special control programmes are organized by WHO.

Animals. Notify internationally (WHO).

Powassan fever

[Powassan encephalitis]

A rare tick-borne viral disease, usually of children, which may occasionally progress to encephalitis. It occurs in Canada and the USA.

The causative agent is the flavivirus complex (Toga-viridae). There is no vaccine.

Reservoir and mode of transmission
The natural reservoir is Ixodes ticks and small wild animals, mainly rodents. Transmission occurs between stages of tick development and through the egg. Domestic animals and humans are infected by tick bites when they enter enzootic areas. Human cases are seasonally related to the period of tick activity. The virus is hazardous to laboratory workers.

Incubation period
Humans.   1–2 weeks.

Animals.   Unknown.

Clinical features
Humans.   There is fever, severe headache and signs of encephalitis.

Animals.   Subclinical.

Pathology
Humans.   There is encephalitis with perivascular cuffing.

Animals.   Unknown.

Special investigations
Humans.   Isolate the virus from brain tissue at post mortem.

Animals.   Serology. Isolate the virus by intracerebral inoculation into mice.

Prognosis
Humans.   It is usually benign, but long-term neurological sequelae are possible.

Animals.   Subclinical only.

Prevention
Humans.   Avoid tick bites and control the tick vector.

Apply strict laboratory safety procedures.

Animals.   Inapplicable.

Treatment
Humans.   Symptomatic therapy.

Animals.   None.

Legislation
Humans.   Acute encephalitis is notifiable in many countries, including the UK and the USA.

Animals.   None.

Q fever

[Query fever, Balkan influenza, Balkan grippe, pneumo-rickettsiosis, abattoir fever]

A febrile rickettsial disease which can cause pneumonia and endocarditis. It occurs worldwide.
    The causative agent is *Coxiella burnetti* (rickettsia).

Reservoir and mode of transmission
Many animals as well as ticks are natural hosts. The reservoir for human infection is usually sheep and cattle. The organisms are abundant in placentae and their fluids and remain viable in dust and litter for months. Infection results from inhalation of contaminated dust, handling infected carcasses or by consumption of contaminated milk or possibly tick bites. The organism is a hazard to laboratory workers.

Incubation period
Humans.   2–4 weeks.

Animals.   Unknown.

Clinical features
Humans.   Fever has acute onset, with muscle pains, severe headache, cough and pneumonitis, hepatitis develops over

a few weeks. Symptoms due to chronic infection may follow, with endocarditis and hepatitis after many years.

Animals.   Abortion may occur (rarely) in sheep and goats.

Pathology
Humans.   Pneumonia sometimes occurs with foci of suppuration and haemorrhage. Foci of chronic inflammatory cells and areas of necrosis occur in the liver. Chronic endocarditis with vegetations on damaged heart valves or prostheses occurs.

Animals.   In cattle the agent localizes in mammary glands, lymph nodes and placenta but no lesions are recorded.

Special investigations
Humans.   Isolation of the causal agent is not usually attempted. A complement fixation test is used for phase-2 antibodies in acute infection and for phase-1 antibodies in chronic infection.

Animals.   Microscopically examine stained smears from cotyledons; serology as for humans.

Prognosis
Humans.   Full recovery is usual in a few weeks and most infections remain subclinical. Chronic endocarditis, particularly in persons with pre-existing valvular disease, is difficult to treat and the case fatality rate may be as high as 60 per cent.

Animals.   Usually subclinical, though abortion can occur.

Prevention
Humans.   Pasteurize milk. Take hygienic precautions in abattoirs and apply animal laboratory hygiene. Apply strict laboratory procedures for handling clinical specimens and cultures.

Animals.   Impracticable.

Treatment
Humans. For acute infection, give tetracycline. For chronic infection, give long-term antibiotic treatment, although the best regimens have yet to be determined. Sometimes surgical removal of the infected heart valve is needed with replacement by a prosthesis.

Animals. Not required.

Vaccination
Humans. Vaccine is available for high-risk groups in certain countries.

Animals. A vaccine has been developed in the USA which is said to be effective in preventing cattle from shedding coxiellae in their milk.

Legislation
Humans. The disease is notifiable in some countries, including Australia, Israel and Italy.

Animals. None.

Queensland tick typhus

[North Queensland tick typhus]

A tick-borne rickettsial fever of Queensland, Australia.
   The causative agent is *Rickettsia australis* (rickettsia). There is no vaccine.

Reservoir and mode of transmission
The organism has been identified from humans and ticks, but serological evidence suggests a reservoir of infection exists in wild marsupials and rodents. Transmission to humans is by tick bite.

Incubation period
Humans. 2–10 days.

Animals. Unknown.

Clinical features
Humans.   Fever lasting up to two weeks has a gradual onset, with headache, malaise and regional lymphadenitis. The skin at the site of the tick bite may develop a papule, leaving a scar. A generalized rash is possible, appearing in the first few days.

Animals.   Unknown.

Pathology
Humans.   Not specific.

Animals.   Unknown.

Special investigations
Humans.   Isolate the organism from blood. Serological tests include the Weil–Felix, complement fixation, microscopic agglutination, indirect haemagglutination and neutralization tests.

Animals.   Not done.

Prognosis
Humans.   It is a benign self-limiting infection.

Animals.   Subclinical as far as known.

Prevention
Humans.   Avoid tick bites. Control the tick vector.

Animals.   Inappropriate.

Treatment
Humans.   Tetracycline therapy.

Animals.   None.

Legislation
Humans.   Typhus (all forms) is notifiable in many countries, including Australia, New Zealand and the UK.

Animals.   None.

Rabies

[Hydrophobia]

A viral infection of the central nervous system. It is usually acquired by humans from animal bites and is invariably fatal in the non-immunized.

Rabies occurs in all continents except Australia and Antarctica. Other rabies-free areas at present include the British Isles, Sweden, New Zealand, Japan, Hawaii, Taiwan, other Pacific islands, and some of the West Indies.

The causative agent is the rabies virus (Rhabdoviridae).

Reservoir and mode of transmission

The virus can infect all warm-blooded animals and birds. Two cycles of transmission are recognized: urban dog rabies, which is now largely confined to the less developed countries, and sylvatic or wildlife rabies which predominates in the USA and much of Europe with various reservoir hosts (e.g. skunks, raccoons and foxes in the USA and Canada, Arctic foxes in the Arctic, mongooses and jackals in Africa, foxes in Europe, blood-feeding bats in South America, other bats in the Americas and Europe). Rabies is fatal in carnivores in which the population density controls the maintenance and spread of infection by biting. Transmission amongst bats is by aerosol inhalation. Most human infections are from bites of domestic carnivores or, in South America, vampire bats. The virus poses a serious hazard to laboratory workers. Person-to-person transmission has resulted from infected corneal transplant grafts.

Incubation period

Humans and animals. This can be from ten days to a year or longer. The incubation period is shorter the nearer the bite is to the head.

Clinical features

Humans. Characteristic symptoms include fever, change in behaviour, anxiety, insomnia, headaches, restlessness, spasmodic contractions of swallowing muscles, especially when offered drinks, developing within a few days to convulsions followed by paralysis and death.

Animals.   Two forms exist, the furious and the paralytic (dumb). Both begin with abnormal behaviour, anorexia followed by agitation and aggression in dogs. Salivation becomes profuse owing to the absence of the swallowing reflex. A tendency to wander is followed by convulsions, paralysis and death. The dumb form goes immediately to paralysis, salivation and death.

Pathology
Humans and animals.   Virus spreads to the CNS via the axoplasm of peripheral nerves and then outwards to salivary glands by a similar route. Specific lesions in the brain include the presence of Negri bodies.

Special investigations
Humans and animals.   Demonstrate the virus in the cornea or brain by immunofluorescence. Do brain histology to demonstrate Negri bodies in stained sections. Isolate virus by intracerebral inoculation of suckling mice.

Prognosis
Humans.   Invariably fatal once symptoms begin.

Animals.   Usually fatal except in bats which are not blood-feeders. Asymptomatic shedding of virus has been reported in Canidae but is very rare.

Prevention
Humans.   In enzootic areas avoid contact with wild animals and promptly cleanse any bite wounds. Specific immunoglobulin is vital as soon as possible after exposure. Pre- and post-exposure vaccination can be given. Apply strict laboratory safety procedures and vaccinate laboratory staff.

Animals.   In enzootic areas vaccinate dogs, cats and cattle. Quarantine all carnivores on importation (six months in Great Britain for carnivores and life-long quarantine for vampire bats). Some countries require vaccination of dogs and cats before import. Vaccinate dogs at land frontiers between enzootic and rabies-free areas.

Treatment

Humans. To prevent development of clinical disease the immediate and vigorous cleansing and disinfection of wounds is vital. This should be followed by infiltration with rabies antiserum coupled with post-exposure immunization using rabies-specific immunoglobulin and vaccine together. There is no specific treatment once rabies has developed, though supportive therapy may help control the distress.

Animals. None. Keep suspected cases under strong confinement and keep under observation for three weeks following contact with infection.

Vaccination

Humans. The vaccine of choice is the human diploid cell vaccine. Pre-exposure vaccination is recommended for those at occupational risk or for travellers to endemic areas likely to be exposed. Post-exposure vaccination in conjunction with specific immunoglobulin is effective.

Animals. Numerous live and attenuated vaccines are available worldwide.

Legislation

Humans. The disease is notifiable in most countries.

Animals. The regulations include notification of suspected cases, slaughter, quarantine, and prohibition of import of dogs and cats. Sometimes there is compulsory vaccination of imported dogs and cats. Muzzling of dogs in public places or in outbreaks may be the rule.

Rickettsialpox

[Vesicular rickettsiosis, Kew Gardens spotted fever]

A rare, mild, benign rickettsial fever in the USSR, Africa and eastern USA. It is transmitted by mites from rodents.

The causative agent is *Rickettsia akari* (rickettsia). There is no vaccine.

Reservoir and mode of transmission
Reservoir hosts are domestic mice and rats, and the mite *Liponyssoides sanguineus*. The organism poses a serious hazard to laboratory staff.

Incubation period
Humans.   10–24 days.

Animals.   Unknown.

Clinical features
Humans.   Illness lasting about a week is associated with an eschar which develops at the site of the mite bite, regional lymphadenopathy and fever. A vesicular rash over the body and limbs develops within 1–4 days.

Animals.   Not known in wild animals. In experimental mice death follows pneumonia.

Pathology
Humans.   There is a vesicular eruption on the skin.

Animals.   Pneumonia occurs in experimental mice.

Special investigations
Humans.   Serology.

Animals.   None.

Prognosis
Humans.   It is a benign, self-limiting illness.

Animals.   Unknown.

Prevention
Humans.   Control rodents and mites. Apply strict laboratory safety procedures.

Animals.   Inappropriate.

Treatment
Humans.   Tetracycline therapy.

Legislation
Humans. All rickettsial infections may be notifiable in some countries (e.g. France and Israel).

Animals. None.

Rift Valley fever

[Enzootic hepatitis]

A severe viral fever which can progress to encephalitis and eye lesions. It affects farm workers and veterinarians in direct contact with infected animals. Large outbreaks have occurred, in southern and central Africa and Egypt.

The causative agent is the Rift Valley fever virus (Bunyaviridae).

Reservoir and mode of transmission
The source of human infection has been sheep, cattle and mosquitoes. The natural reservoir is not yet defined. Human infection is probably from contamination of wounds and abrasions, and possibly from inhalation of aerosols and from mosquito bites. The virus poses a serious hazard to laboratory workers.

Incubation period
Humans. 3–7 days.

Animals. 1–3 days.

Clinical features
Humans. Fever (which may be biphasic) has a sudden onset, with severe headache, muscle and joint pains and photophobia. In a small proportion of cases there are haemorrhages, liver necrosis, encephalitis and retinitis.

Animals. Rapid death after fever occurs in lambs. In cattle abortion and diarrhoea occur.

Pathology
Humans. Features sometimes include encephalitis, retinal exudates and generalized haemorrhages.

Animals.   Liver lesions predominate, with areas of necrosis. Widespread haemorrhages occur.

Special investigations
Humans.   Isolate virus from the blood. Serological tests include the neutralization test.

Animals.   Isolate virus in mice or tissue culture.

Prognosis
Humans.   There may be high mortality in epidemics. In survivors convalescence is prolonged but usually complete. There may be permanent damage to the eye.

Animals.   Mortality is generally low in animals, but the disease is highly fatal in newborn lambs.

Prevention
Humans.   Control mosquitoes. Dispose of infected animals effectively. Apply strict laboratory safety procedures and vaccinate laboratory staff.

Animals.   Remove stock from the mosquito environment, or bring it into stables.

Treatment
Humans.   Symptomatic therapy.

Animals.   None.

Vaccination
Humans.   Formol inactivated vaccine has been used for veterinarians and laboratory workers in enzootic areas.

Animals.   Recommended in enzootic areas.

Legislation
Humans.   In some countries the disease is notifiable specifically, and as acute encephalitis in other countries including the UK, the USA and New Zealand.

Animals.   None.

Ringworm

[Dermatophytosis, dermatomycosis, tinea, trichophytosis, microsporosis]

A fungal skin disease acquired by contact with infectious humans or animals. It occurs worldwide.

In zoonotic ringworm the pathogens include various species of Trichophyton and Microsporum, mainly *T. mentagrophytes, T. verrucosum* and *M. canis* (pathogenic fungi).

Reservoir and mode of transmission

Trichophyton infection in humans is acquired from horses and cattle, Microsporum infection from dogs. Fungal spores remain viable for long periods on carrier animals, harness, tackle, etc. Transmission occurs by contact with animals. Person-to-person transmission is rare. Animals serve as reservoirs of infection, generating spores which contaminate the environment.

Incubation period

Humans.   4–14 days.

Animals.   1–4 weeks.

Clinical features

Humans.   Ring-shaped, scaly and crusty skin lesions spread on the scalp (with loss of hair), or other parts of the body.

Animals.   Lesions are common in housed cattle and calves. They appear as grey-white plaques on the head and neck and gradually enlarge.

Pathology

Humans and animals.   Varying severity of dermatitis occurs with local loss of hair. The fungal hyphae grow in the stratum corneum and must keep pace with the rate of skin growth to induce a lesion. Deeper invasion produces a mild inflammatory reaction which increases in severity with the development of hypersensitivity.

Special investigations
Humans.   Identify the organism in skin scrapings.

Animals.   Microscopically examine scrapings from the edge of a lesion for fungal spores after clearing with potassium or sodium hydroxide. Identify species of fungus by culture. Examine cats, which often show no lesions, under an ultraviolet light fitted with a Wood's filter to reveal infection by Microsporum, many species of which fluoresce.

Prognosis
Humans.   Chronic benign infection is usual, which may become secondarily infected.

Animals.   Although prolonged this is a non-fatal self-limiting skin disease.

Prevention
Humans.   Avoid direct contact with infected animals and wash hands after contact. Treat early to prevent person-to-person spread.

Animals.   Give farm animals adequate nourishment and sunlight. Vaccinate, isolate and treat all affected animals; disinfect grooming tools and equipment using formaldehyde and buildings using sodium hydroxide.

Treatment
Humans.   Oral griseofulvin; topical antifungal agents.

Animals.   Oral griseofulvin for severe, extensive lesions.

Vaccination
Humans.   None.

Animals.   Immunization of farm animals using a live spore vaccine is successfully practised in some European countries.

Legislation
Humans and animals.   None.

Rocio viral encephalitis

An epidemic viral encephalitis which occurs in localized parts of Brazil. It affects mainly outdoor workers and is transmitted by mosquitoes from wild birds.

The causative agent is the Rocio virus (Togaviridae). There is no vaccine.

Reservoir and mode of transmission
Serological evidence exists of a reservoir in wild birds. Transmission is presumed to be by mosquito bites. Person-to-person transmission does not appear to occur. The virus poses a serious hazard to laboratory workers.

Incubation period
Humans. 1–2 weeks.

Animals. Unknown.

Clinical features
Humans. Fever has a sudden onset, with malaise, headache and neck stiffness. Neurological symptoms include confusion and cerebellar motor dysfunction.

Animals. Unknown.

Pathology
Humans. Focal haemorrhages occur in the brain stem and cerebellum.

Animals. Unknown.

Special investigations
Humans. Isolate virus from the brain at post mortem. Serological tests include haemagglutination inhibition, complement fixation and neutralization tests.

Animals. None.

Prognosis
Humans. The case fatality rate is about 5 per cent. Residual neurological defects are common.

Animals.   Unknown.

Prevention
Humans.   Avoid outbreak areas. Apply strict laboratory safety procedures.

Animals.   None.

Treatment
Humans.   Symptomatic therapy.

Animals.   None.

Legislation
Humans.   The disease is notifiable during epidemics in Brazil. In other countries imported cases may be notifiable as acute encephalitis.

Animals.   None.

Rocky Mountain spotted fever

[American tick typhus, spotted fever, tick-borne typhus fever]

A severe tick-borne rickettsial infection, occurring mainly in spring, throughout the USA, Canada and some Central and South American countries.
  The causative agent is *Rickettsia rickettsi* (rickettsia).

Reservoir and mode of transmission
The natural reservoirs are ticks (wood-tick *Dermacenter andersoni* in western USA areas and the dog tick *D. canabilis* in the eastern USA), dogs, rodents and other animals. Most rickettsias are obligate intracellular parasites of the gut cells of invertebrates and can only survive briefly outside living cells. Transmission is by tick bite to humans, dogs, rodents and other animals. Crushed ticks or mites and their faeces may infect through broken skin. Infection is maintained by passage through the invertebrate egg and from stage to stage in ticks. Transmission from tick bite

occurs only after several hours of attachment. The organism poses a serious hazard to laboratory workers.

Incubation period

Humans. 2–14 days.

Animals. Infection is subclinical in most natural hosts.

Clinical features

Humans. Fever has a sudden onset, with chills, headache, severe muscle pains, photophobia and meningism for four weeks. A red, morbilliform rash develops within 3–5 days of onset of fever and with haemorrhages spreading on limbs. Enlarged liver and spleen, myocarditis, renal tubular necrosis and bronchopneumonia occur.

Animals. Subclinical only.

Pathology

Humans. Damage to endothelial cells of blood vessels by invasion of rickettsias causes thrombi and haemorrhages. Focal liver necrosis, haemorrhages in genitalia and gangrene of the scrotum may occur.

Animals. Unknown.

Special investigations

Humans. Isolate rickettsias from blood. Serological tests include the Weil–Felix, complement fixation, indirect haemagglutination and microagglutination tests.

Animals. Demonstrate the organism in stained blood or tissue smears. Serology is as for humans.

Prognosis

Humans. The case fatality rate in untreated cases is 15–20 per cent, but with prompt treatment is about 5 per cent. Severe complications may result from secondary infection and gangrene.

Animals. The course of infection in animals is unknown but is probably mild or inapparent.

Prevention
Humans.   Control tick vectors. Avoid tick bites. Carefully look for and remove any attached ticks. Apply strict laboratory safety procedures.

Animals.   Control ticks.

Treatment
Humans.   Tetracyclines, chloramphenicol.

Animals.   None.

Vaccination
Humans.   Killed vaccine has been used for persons at high risk but is not now available.

Animals.   None.

Legislation
Humans.   Notifiable is required in the USA and some other countries.

Animals.   None.

Russian spring summer encephalitis

[Tick-borne   encephalitis,   Far   Eastern   tick-borne encephalitis, Central European tick-borne encephalitis]

A severe viral encephalitis in the USSR and Europe, transmitted by tick bites. Outbreaks have occurred from consumption of raw milk.

The causative agents are tick-borne encephalitis viruses (Togaviridae).

Reservoir and mode of transmission
The natural reservoir is wild and domestic animals, especially rodents, goats, sheep and cattle and Ixodes ticks. Transmission to humans is by tick bites, consumption of unpasteurized milk and by laboratory accidents.

Incubation period
Humans. 1–2 weeks.

Animals. Unknown.

Clinical features
Humans. Fever (which may be biphasic) has a sudden onset, with severe headache, anorexia, nausea and vomiting, visual disturbances, and meningism. Neurological symptoms include fits, paralysis and coma. Death or recovery usually occurs within one week.

Animals. Unknown.

Pathology
Humans. Meningoencephalitis. Leucopenia is characteristic.

Animals. Unknown.

Special investigations
Humans. Isolate virus from blood; serology.

Animals. None.

Prognosis
Humans. The case fatality rate is up to 30 per cent. Residual paralysis and neurological defects are common, and convalescence may be prolonged.

Animals. Unknown.

Prevention
Humans. Avoid tick-infested areas and tick bites. Heat-treat milk. Apply maximum laboratory safety procedures.

Animals. None attempted.

Treatment
Humans. Symptomatic therapy.

Animals. None.

Vaccination
Humans. Experimental at present.

Animals. None.

Legislation
Humans. Acute encephalitis is notifiable in many countries, including the UK and the USA.

Animals. None.

Salmonellosis

[Salmonella food poisoning, enteric paratyphosis]

A common bacterial cause of food-poisoning worldwide.

Over 1800 food-poisoning serotypes of salmonella (bacterium) exist. The prevalence of individual serotypes constantly changes.

Reservoir and mode of transmission

Salmonellas are common commensals of all animals and birds and are excreted in faeces. Host-adapted strains may cause serious illness (e.g. *S. dublin* in cattle, *S. pulorum* in chickens), but most human food-poisoning salmonellas do not cause clinical signs in animals. The main reservoirs for human infection are poultry, cattle, sheep and pigs. Infection in animals is maintained by recycling slaughterhouse waste as animal feed, faecal oral spread and faecal contamination of hatching eggs. Transmission occurs when organisms, introduced into the kitchen in poultry carcasses, meat or unpasteurized milk, multiply in food owing to inadequate cooking, cross-contamination of cooked foods and inadequate storage. Person-to-person spread in common in institutions such as hospitals.

Incubation period

Humans. 12–72 hours.

Animals. 1–5 days.

Clinical features

Humans. The presence and severity of symptoms depends on the infecting dose. Typically there is watery diarrhoea for about ten days, possibly leading to dehydration, with abdominal pain and low-grade fever. Septicaemia and abscess formation are rare.

Animals. Subclinical infection is common and many animals may be intermittent or persistent carriers. However, cows may suffer with fever, diarrhoea and abortion. Calves undergo epizootic outbreaks of diarrhoea with high mortality. In pigs, fever and diarrhoea are less common than in cattle. Infected sheep, goats and poultry usually show no signs of infection.

Pathology

Humans. Enteritis is a feature. Extra-intestinal infection may cause abscesses.

Animals. Penetration of the infection into the mucosa is followed by inflammation, especially ileitis, progressing to inflamed mesenteric lymph nodes in the mesentery, possibly progressing to septicaemia and pneumonia especially in calves. Dehydration and rapid loss of weight are due to stimulation of chloride excretion and inhibition of sodium absorption. Abortion in cattle is caused by massive proliferation of salmonella in the placenta leading to placental necrosis.

Special investigations

Humans. Isolate salmonella from faeces and suspected foods using selective media followed by serotyping and, if appropriate, phage typing.

Animals. Culture faeces, post-mortem tissues and foods of animal origin. Serological tests are of limited value as many non-infected animals have titres from past infections.

Prognosis

Humans. Usually only a self-limiting illness occurs. Deaths from dehydration or septicaemia are rare and occur usually in infants, or debilitated or elderly patients.

Animals. There is abortion in cattle and endometritis with temporary infertility. In calves, dehydration and septicaemia may lead to death.

Prevention
Humans. Educate food handlers in good kitchen hygiene. Ensure thorough cooking of meat, refrigerate cooked foods and prevent cross-contamination. Pasteurize all milk. Ensure personal hygiene. Reduce contamination of poultry carcasses at abattoirs. Irradiation of meat and other foods before purchase will reduce contamination.

Animals. This is difficult and often impractical because there are many sources of infection. Principles of control include the following: maintain closed herds and flocks; keep animals in small groups; purchase replacements direct from the farm of origin; avoid mixing animals from different sources; sterilize ingredients of animal feed; provide mains drinking water for grazing livestock; prevent access of wild birds and rodents to animal houses; completely destock animals and thoroughly cleanse and disinfect housing between batches; monitor poultry breeding stock and remove excretors; disinfect hatching eggs and fumigate incubators.

Treatment
Humans. Undertake fluid replacement therapy with antibiotics in severe cases. Antibiotics are said to increase the duration of excretion of salmonellas.

Animals. Treatment with antibiotics and sulphonamides immediately diarrhoea and fever occur reduces mortality but is contraindicated in healthy carriers in which treatment may prolong the carrier state.

Vaccination
Humans. None.

Animals. Vaccines are available against *S. dublin* and *S. typhimurium* in calves. A live vaccine prepared from a rough strain of *S. dublin* gives good protection in calves against both *S. dublin* and *S. typhimurium*.

Legislation
Humans. The disease is notifiable specifically in the USA, Australia, New Zealand and several European countries, or as food-poisoning as in the UK.

Animals. Notification of infection in food animals is obligatory in some countries, including the UK, with statutory sampling of animal protein for animal feed. Heat-treatment of waste food applies in the UK. A slaughter policy is claimed in Luxembourg, Germany and Czechoslovakia.

Scabies

[Scabiosis, mange, acariasis, sarcoptic itch]

A skin disease caused worldwide by mites.

Sarcoptes scabei is the usual agent of human scabies. *S. ovis, S. equi* and *Notoedres cati* can occasionally infect humans (Arthropoda). There is no vaccine.

Reservoir and mode of transmission
The mite is transmitted by direct or indirect contact. It can survive for several days off the host. Cross-species transmission is not common.

Incubation period
Humans. For a first infection the period is 2–6 weeks; for a subsequent infection (after sensitization) it is 1–4 days.

Animals. Variable.

Clinical features
Humans. The disease usually appears on the skin between fingers, at the groin and beneath breasts. Eggs deposited in the epidermis hatch after 3–4 days and larvae excavate new tunnels. An intense irritation is provoked, causing itching of inflamed tracks with excoriation and secondary spread.

Animals. Intense itching causes scratching and spread of infection. Characteristic papules and vesicles form.

Pathology

Humans. The mite tunnels in the epidermis. Intense irritation leads to scratching, spread of infection and possibly purulent secondary infection.

Animals. The tunnelling mites induce allergic sensitization with vesicle formation. The skin thickens and there is loss of hair.

Special investigations

Humans and animals. Examine deep skin scrapings microscopically for mites after clearing with potassium or sodium hydroxide.

Prognosis

Humans. The disease responds well to treatment but repeated infection is likely in crowded, unhygienic conditions.

Animals. Although a non-fatal skin disease, it can prove intractable to treatment in dogs.

Prevention

Humans. Prompt treatment is necessary. Isolate infected persons. Disinfect clothes and bedding.

Animals. Give adequate nutrition and good hygiene. Treat sows three times at weekly intervals before farrowing to prevent infection of the newborn. Quarantine or prohibit imports of live animals from affected countries.

Treatment

Humans. Use topical applications of benzene hexachloride, benzyl benzoate or monosulfiram. Bath and wear clean clothes regularly.

Animals. Thoroughly soak the skin of all animals in an affected group with insecticide (e.g. lindane or organophosphates) applied as a wash, dip or spray, and repeat on two or three occasions at intervals of 10–14 days. Disinfect or rest buildings for three weeks. In small animals benzyl benzoate may be painted on the lesions and allowed to dry, or tetraethylthiuram monosulphide or carbarol applied as a wash. Oral medications are also available for small animals and ivermectin for cattle as a subcutaneous injection.

Legislation
Humans. The disease is notifiable in some European countries.

Animals. The disease is notifiable, with compulsory treatment in sheep, horses and cattle, in many countries.

Schistosomiasis

[Bilharzia, bilharziasis]

A systemic water-borne flatworm infection which can lead to liver failure and neurological damage.

The causative agents are Schistosoma species, including *Shistosoma mansoni* and *S. haematobium* for which humans are the reservoir; and *S. japonicum* which is zoonotic (Trematoda). There is no vaccine.

S. mansoni occurs in Africa, South America and some Caribbean islands; *S. haematobium* in Africa and the Middle East; and *S. japonicum* in China, Japan, the Philippines and South East Asia.

Reservoir and mode of transmission
S. japonicum infects cattle, water buffalo, horses, dogs, cats, rodents and monkeys (*S. bovis* and *S. mattheii*: sheep and cattle). Intermediate hosts are species of snails (Biomphalaria and Bulinus). Cercariae in contaminated water penetrate human skin, especially in irrigated fields or rivers. In the body the parasite migrates via the liver to the superior mesenteric vein where maturation takes place in about six weeks. Eggs are disseminated throughout the body via the blood, released into the intestinal lumen and excreted. In water miracidia develop and penetrate the snail, which in turn excretes cercariae into the water.

Incubation period
Humans. *S. japonicum* incubates for 4–6 weeks prior to acute symptoms.

Animals.   Variable.

Clinical features
Humans.   Penetration of larvae through the skin causes an itchy rash (this is the only symptom, 'swimmer's itch', from the animal and bird schistosomes which do not invade in humans). With *S. japonicum* acute symptoms include fever, abdominal pain, cough, weight loss, diarrhoea and dysentery. Chronic infection may result in symptoms months to years later, with enlarged liver and spleen, cirrhosis, ascites, and fits due to cerebral involvement.

Animals.   Abdominal pain, diarrhoea, anaemia and emaciation occur. Haematuria is said to be a feature in cattle.

Pathology
Humans and animals.   With heavy infection, penetration of the parasite through the skin gives local dermatitis followed by pneumonitis when the parasites reach the lung. The deposition of ova provokes the growth of small multiple granulomata throughout the body. Eventually intestinal and hepatic fibroses develop. Eosinophilia is prominent.

Special investigations
Humans.   Identify eggs in faeces or biopsy tissue. Serological tests include indirect haemagglutination, ELISA, indirect immunofluorescence and complement fixation tests.

Animals.   Examine faeces for fluke eggs.

Prognosis
Humans.   Chronic infection results in portal cirrhosis, liver failure and CNS lesions.

Animals.   Spontaneous recovery occurs from acute intestinal schistosomiasis. The chronic hepatic syndrome may occasionally lead to death from congestive heart failure. Treatment may result in embolism of hepatic portal veins and hepatic failure.

Prevention
Humans.   Sanitary care is needed with disposal of faeces and urine. Avoid skin exposure to contaminated water. Treat cases promptly. Destroy snails and their habitat. Gloves should be worn by laboratory workers.

Animals. Control the snail intermediate host using molluscicides. Provide piped drinking water and keep water troughs clean. Dispose of sewage with proper processing.

Treatment
Humans.   Praziquantel.

Animals.   Tartar emetic, antimosan and stibophen are effective in cattle, lucanthone and trichlorophon in cattle and sheep, hycanthone and niridazole in sheep.

Legislation
Humans.   The disease is notifiable in some endemic areas and some other countries, including New Zealand.

Animals.   None.

Scrub typhus

[Tsutsugamushi disease, mite-borne typhus fever, Japanese river fever]

A severe, sporadic, rickettsial disease transmitted by mites from rodents. It occurs in central, eastern and south eastern Asia in small, well-defined areas.
    The causative agent is *Rickettsia tsutsugamushi* (rickettsia).

Reservoir and mode of transmission
The reservoirs are larvae of trombiculid mites and various species of rodent and insectivores. Animal hosts may not be essential to maintenance of the cycle. Transmission is by the bite of mite larvae. Nymphs and adults do not feed on vertebrates. Infection cycles amongst mites and small animals. Humans are accidental hosts. Transovarial

transmission occurs in the mite. The organism poses a serious hazard to laboratory workers.

Incubation period
Humans.   4–21 days.

Animals.   Unknown.

Clinical features
Humans.   An eschar develops at the site of the bite, with regional lymphadenitis, sudden onset of fever which lasts 2–3 weeks, severe headache, lymphadenopathy, rash appearing after about five days and persisting for up to one week, cough, conjunctivitis and CNS signs.

Animals.   Disease is very mild and usually subclinical.

Pathology
Humans.   Inflammation and necrosis occur at the site of the eschar. The endothelium of blood vessels is damaged, resulting in thrombosis and haemorrhage. Focal necrosis occurs in liver and spleen.

Animals.   Probably none.

Special investigations
Humans.   Isolate the organism from blood. Serological tests include Weil–Felix and complement fixation tests.

Animals.   None.

Prognosis
Humans.   The case fatality rises to 60 per cent if untreated.

Animals.   Infection is mild or inapparent.

Prevention
Humans.   Avoid mite bites and control mite vectors. Consider the use of doxycycline for chemoprophylaxis in persons likely to be exposed. Apply strict laboratory safety procedures.

Animals.   Impracticable.

Treatment
Humans.   Tetracyclines.

Animals.   None.

Vaccination
Humans.   None.

Animals.   Inappropriate.

Legislation
Humans.   'Typhus' is notifiable in some countries, including the UK, Australia and New Zealand.

Animals.   None.

Semliki Forest virus infection

A mosquito-borne viral infection not yet known to cause symptoms, although the virus appears to be widely distributed in Africa.

The causative agent is the Semliki Forest virus (Togaviridae). There is no vaccine.

Reservoir and mode of transmission
Virus has been isolated from a wide range of animals and birds as well as mosquitoes. Transmission is thought to be from mosquito bites and laboratory accidents. Serological evidence exists of widespread human infection in the endemic areas.

Incubation period
Humans.   Uncertain.

Animals.   Unknown.

Clinical features
Humans.   Asymptomatic.

Animals.   Unknown, but probably subclinical.

Pathology
Humans and animals.   None.

Special investigations
Humans.   Serology.

Animals.   Impracticable.

Prognosis
Humans.   No clinical illness yet reported.

Animals.   Subclinical.

Prevention
Humans.   Apply laboratory safety procedures.

Animals.   Inappropriate.

Treatment
Humans and animals.   None.

Legislation
Humans and animals.   None.

St Louis encephalitis

[Type C lethargic encephalitis]

A viral encephalitis transmitted by mosquitoes from wild birds. It occurs sporadically and in epidemics, in North and Central America and the West Indies.

The causative agent is the St Louis encephalitis virus (Togaviridae). There is no vaccine.

Reservoir and mode of transmission
The natural reservoirs are birds and mosquitoes. Mammals can be infected and bats may play a part in the over-

wintering of St Louis virus. Humans are an accidental host infected by mosquito bites and in laboratory accidents.

Incubation period
Humans.   5–15 days.

Animals.   Subclinical.

Clinical features
Humans.   Usually only a mild fever occurs for a few days, but severe fever and convulsions may develop. Clinical symptoms are more severe in the elderly and very mild in children.

Animals.   Subclinical, though viraemia occurs.

Pathology
Humans.   There is possibly encephalitis with perivascular cuffing and brain haemorrhages.

Animals.   Unknown, but probably none.

Special investigations
Humans.   Serological tests include complement fixation, haemagglutination inhibition and neutralization tests. Virus isolation from blood and cerebrospinal fluid is seldom achieved.

Animals.   None.

Prognosis
Humans.   It is often a benign self-limiting infection, but the case fatality rate in outbreaks may be up to 30 per cent in humans over 50 years of age.

Animals.   Subclinical.

Prevention
Humans.   Control the mosquito vector and prevent mosquito bites. Apply strict laboratory safety procedures.

Animals.   Vector control.

Treatment
Humans.   Symptomatic therapy.

Animals.   None.

Legislation
Humans.   'Acute encephalitis' is notifiable in many countries, including the UK, USA and New Zealand.

Animals.   None.

Streptobacillary fever

[Rat bite fever, Haverhill fever, epidemic arthritic erythema, sodoku]

A relapsing bacterial fever with arthropathy, acquired from infected rat bites and contaminated milk and water. It occurs worldwide.

The causative agents are *Streptobacillus moniliformis* and *Spirillum minus* (sodoku) (bacterium). There is no vaccine.

Reservoir and mode of transmission

The natural reservoir is rats which excrete organisms in their urine and in saliva. Human infection is acquired from rat bites, ingestion of contaminated milk or water, or by handling infected animals or contaminated articles.

Incubation period

Humans.   Streptobacillary fever: 3–10 days; sodoku: 5–30 days.

Animals.   Subclinical.

Clinical features

Humans.   With *S. moniliformis* infection there is fever for a few days, with headache, malaise, nausea, migratory joint pains, erythematous maculopapular rash on hands and feet, photophobia, pharyngitis. Short relapses may occur for several weeks, with possibly endocarditis. With *Spirillum minus* infection there is ulceration at the site of the bite, regional lymphadenitis, relapsing fever, malaise, and a purple rash on chest and arms.

Animals.   Subclinical.

Pathology
Humans.   Not characteristic. Complications have included endocarditis, polyarthritis and lymphadenopathy.

Animals.   None.

Special investigations
Humans and animals.   Isolate *S. moniliformis* from blood. Demonstrate *S. minus* in blood smears and isolate by animal inoculation.

Prognosis
Humans.   The case fatality rate is up to 10 per cent in untreated cases.

Animals.   Subclinical.

Prevention
Humans.   Control rats. Heat-treat milk. Protect water supplies from contamination.

Animals.   None.

Treatment
Humans.   Penicillin is usually effective in early cases.

Animals.   None.

Legislation
Humans.   The disease is not usually notifiable.

Animals.   None.

Streptococcosis

[*Streptococcus suis* infection, *S. zooepidemicus* infection]

A number of unusual bacterial infections acquired from

occupational exposure. They occasionally cause severe disease.

The causative agents are various streptococci species, including *Streptococcus suis* and *S. zooepidemicus* (bacterium). There is no vaccine.

S. suis infection has been reported from Europe, including the UK, Brazil, the USA and Australia, and is probably present in all the major pig-producing countries. *S. zooepidemicus* infection of humans has been reported from Britain and Rumania.

Reservoir and mode of transmission

Pigs are the reservoir of *S. suis*. Many carry the organism in their tonsils and noses. Occasionally the infection spreads to the meninges and joints. Humans are infected handling the infected meat. *S. zooepidemicus* infection has occurred in persons in direct contact with domestic animals and from drinking raw milk.

Incubation period

Humans.   Uncertain, but probably a few days.

Animals.   Variable.

Clinical features

Humans.   *S. suis* causes fever and occasionally meningitis. *S. zooepidemicus* may cause upper respiratory tract symptoms, cervical adenitis, pneumonia, endocarditis and nephritis.

Animals.   *S. suis* epizootics may occur in pigs with high mortality, heralded by signs of meningitis including depression, fever, incoordination and paralysis. More usually the disease is subclinical. *S. zooepidemicus* may cause mastitis in cattle.

Pathology

Humans.   There are occasional abscesses and streptococcal meningitis.

Animals.   *S. suis* causes meningoencephalitis. Abscesses in the retropharyngeal and cervical lymph nodes are common in subclinical cases. Suppurative arthritis may occur.

Special investigations
Humans. Isolate the organism from throat swabs, cerebrospinal fluid and blood.

Animals. Isolate the organism at post mortem examination. Fluorescent antibody tests may be applied to tissue and exudate smears.

Prognosis
Humans. A fatality rate of 8 per cent has been reported for *S. suis*, with residual deafness in a high proportion of survivors.

Animals. Mortality may reach 50 per cent despite treatment in pigs showing nervous signs. Polyarthritis is a chronic sequel in some cases.

Prevention
Humans. Exercise extreme care in handling pig meat. Dress all wounds to avoid contamination. Pasteurize milk.

Animals. Inspect herds frequently and treat clinical cases. Provide adequate space, ventilation and freedom from stress. In-feed medication of the herd at times of risk will reduce cases but not eradicate infection.

Treatment
Humans. Antibiotic (penicillin) therapy.

Animals. Antibiotic (e.g. penicillin) injections, removal from the group and supportive measures bring about complete recovery if applied early.

Legislation
Humans. Acute meningitis is notifiable in many countries, including the UK.

Animals. None.

Strongyloidiasis

[Strongyloidosis]

A chronic roundworm infection transmitted by direct contact with faeces. It occurs worldwide, in warm, wet regions.

The causative agents are *Strongyloides stercoralis* and *S. fuelleborni* (Nematoda). There is no vaccine.

Reservoir and mode of transmission

Reservoir hosts of *S. stercoralis* are ducks, dogs and cats, and of *S. fuelleborni* non-human primates. Humans are infected by skin penetration of larvae. These are then carried by the blood to the lungs and thence up the trachea to the alimentary tract. Eggs are shed in the faeces which develop into larvae in soil, thus completing the cycle. Autoinfection can occur.

Incubation period

Humans.   2–4 weeks.

Animals.   Subclinical, except in young dogs and cats.

Clinical features

Humans.   Skin inflammation and pruritis at the site of penetration of larvae may be followed by fever, cough, haemoptysis, mucoid diarrhoea and abdominal pain. Malabsorption and gastrointestinal bleeding are possible. Hyperinfection and disseminated forms of larval migration give severe symptoms.

Animals.   Young dogs and cats have thin skins which allow massive infection to penetrate, giving severe dermatitis, inappetence, coughing and even bronchopneumonia. Vomiting occurs, as does severe dermatitis during the period of larval penetration.

Pathology

Humans.   Small papules occur where larvae penetrate the skin. Pneumonitis and bronchopneumonia can occur. Intestinal infection produces enteritis leading to ulceration. Dead and dying aberrant larvae can induce foci of inflammation throughout the body, and eosinophilia.

Animals. Alopecia and bronchopneumonia occur, followed by dehydration, anaemia and sometimes death.

Special investigations
Humans and animals. Examine fresh faeces for motile larvae (*S. stercoralis*) or embryonated eggs (*S. fuelleborni*).

Prognosis
Humans. Chronic infection may persist for years, even after moving from an endemic area, owing to autoinfection. The hyperinfection syndrome and disseminated infection may prove fatal.

Animals. Subclinical or self-limiting disease usually occurs, in dogs and cats. It is rarely fatal.

Prevention
Humans. Prevent exposure by wearing shoes. Dispose of faeces with proper sanitary care. Use good personal hygiene to prevent autoinfection through perianal skin.

Animals. Ensure proper sewage disposal. Provide clean, dry housing for domestic animals.

Treatment
Humans. Thiabendazole and mebendazole.

Animals. Thiabendazole is the drug of choice.

Legislation
Humans and animals. None.

Swine vesicular disease

A transient viral disease of pigs causing vesicular lesions around the mouth and feet. Its main importance is the possibility of confusion with foot and mouth disease. Human infection rarely results from occupational exposure.

An apparently new disease spreading rapidly throughout the world, it was first isolated in Italy, then in Hong Kong,

Japan, Malta and many European countries. It is probably present in all major pig-producing countries.

The causative agent is the swine vesicular disease virus (Picornaviridae).

Reservoir and mode of transmission

The reservoir is pigs. The virus has unusual chemical and physical resistance and may remain infective in the environment for months. It is easily spread mechanically on equipment or in feed. Infection is through minor abrasions in the skin, especially of the feet, from virus excreted in oral and nasal secretions, faeces and vesicle fluid. Air-borne spread is not a feature. Infected pigs shed virus from shortly before onset of signs for three weeks and, exceptionally, up to three months afterwards.

Incubation period

Humans.   Uncertain.

Animals.   2–14 days.

Clinical features

Humans.   It is an influenza-like illness lasting 1–5 weeks.

Animals.   In pigs there is transient fever, followed by the development of vesicles around the hooves with casting off of claws. Some vesicles may appear on the snout or in the mouth.

Pathology

Humans.   Uncertain.

Animals.   Vesicles follow a brief period of viraemia. Lesions in the brain have been seen but usually without clinical signs.

Special investigations

Humans.   Isolate the virus from nasal and pharyngeal secretions.

Animals.   Serology. Demonstrate the viral antigen in vesicle material by a fluorescent antibody test or with the aid of tissue culture.

Prognosis
Humans.   It is a self-limiting illness.

Animals.   Usually mild, followed by complete recovery.

Prevention
Humans.   Exercise care in handling infective pigs and material.

Animals.   Quarantine imported pigs, prohibit imports from affected countries, cook waste intended for pig feeding. Slaughter policy is applied in outbreaks with movement restrictions in the affected area.

Treatment
Humans.   Symptomatic therapy.

Animals.   Inappropriate.

Vaccination
Humans.   None.

Animals.   An inactivated vaccine has been used in France.

Legislation
Humans.   None.

Animals.   Because of the similarity to foot and mouth disease a slaughter policy is adopted in many countries.

Tahyna virus infection

A benign viral fever of children which may occasionally progress to meningoencephalitis. It occurs in Central Europe and Africa.

The causative agent is the tahyna virus (Bunyaviridae). There is no vaccine.

Reservoir and mode of transmission
The natural reservoir is wild animals and mosquitoes. Transmission is by mosquito bite, from July to September, in endemic areas of Europe.

Incubation period
Humans. Uncertain.

Animals. Unknown.

Clinical features
Humans. Usually there is fever, headache, nausea, pharyngitis and conjunctivitis for a few days, and rarely bronchopneumonia and meningoencephalitis occur.

Animals. Unknown, but presumably subclinical.

Pathology
Humans. Not specific, but includes aseptic meningitis and encephalitis.

Animals. Unknown.

Special investigations
Humans. Serological tests include complement fixation, haemagglutination inhibition and neutralization tests.

Animals. Unknown.

Prognosis
Humans. It is usually a benign, self-limiting illness.

Animals. Unknown.

Prevention
Humans. Control mosquito vectors and avoid their bites.

Animals. None.

Treatment
Humans. Symptomatic therapy.

Animals. None.

Legislation
Humans. Acute encephalitis is notifiable in many countries, including the UK and the USA.

Animals. None.

Tanapox

A rare, benign, viral infection occurring in Kenya, in out-breaks.

The causative agent is the tanapox virus (Poxviridae). There is no vaccine.

Reservoir and mode of transmission

The reservoir is believed to be monkeys, with mechanical transmission to humans by mosquitoes and laboratory accidents.

Incubation period

Humans. Uncertain.

Animals. Unknown.

Clinical features

Humans. There is fever for a few days, with headache and prostration and a single skin vesicle.

Animals. Lesions occur primarily on the face, consisting of raised areas with a central scab.

Pathology

Humans. Cytoplasmic inclusions are seen in skin lesions.

Animals. Papules ulcerate, scab and heal.

Special investigations

Humans and animals. Identify the virus by electron microscopy of skin scrapings. Isolate the virus from lesions.

Prognosis

Humans. It is a mild self-limiting illness.

Animals. The pox lesions heal uneventfully. Even severe lesions regress in 6–8 weeks.

Prevention
Humans.   Avoid mosquito bites. Apply laboratory safety procedures.

Animals.   Protect laboratory monkeys from mosquitoes.

Treatment
Humans.   Symptomatic therapy.

Animals.   None.

Legislation
Humans and animals.   None.

Thelaziasis

[Conjunctival spirurosis]

A painful roundworm infection of the eye. It occurs in India, Burma, China, the Americas and Australia.

The causative agents are *Thelazia callipaeda, T. californiensis* and *T. rhodesi* (Nematoda). There is no vaccine.

Reservoir and mode of transmission
Reservoirs are several species of domestic and wild mammals. The adult worm lodges in the conjunctivae. Intermediate hosts include various species of flies. Flies ingest the eggs and larvae by sucking secretions from the corner of the eye. These larvae develop in stages and eventually migrate to the proboscis where they are released when the fly again feeds on ocular secretions.

Incubation period
Humans.   Uncertain.

Animals.   Unknown.

Clinical features
Humans and animals.   The condition consists of severe and painful conjunctivitis with lachrymation.

Pathology
Humans. There is possible scarring of the cornea in severe cases.

Animals. There is mild to severe conjunctivitis, with opacity and ulceration of the cornea in severe cases.

Special investigations
Humans and animals. Examine the contents of a conjunctival sac for the worms.

Prognosis
Humans and animals. Symptoms subside when worms are removed.

Prevention
Humans and animals. Ensure good personal hygiene, and control flies.

Treatment
Humans and animals. Surgically remove worms from the conjunctival sac.

Legislation
Humans and animals. None.

Toxocariasis

[Visceral larva migrans, larval granulomatosis, ocular larva migrans]

A common roundworm infection of dogs and cats, acquired by humans worldwide in childhood by ingesting eggs. Symptomatic disease is rare but occurs particularly in children subject to pica.

The causative agents are *Toxocara canis* and *T. cati* (*T. mystax*) (Nematoda). There is no vaccine.

Reservoir and mode of transmission
Reservoir hosts are dogs and cats. Eggs excreted in faeces require a maturation period in soil. Eggs hatch in the intestine and larvae penetrate the intestine wall to enter the blood vessels. In puppies less than five weeks old, larvae

migrate to the intestines via the lungs and complete their maturation. Dormant larvae in adults reactivate during pregnancy and migrate to the placenta and mature in puppies, or may infect puppies via milk. Larvae excreted in faeces by puppies may mature in the bitch once ingested. Humans are infected when eggs from contaminated soil, grass, etc., are ingested. Children with pica are at greatest risk.

Incubation period
Humans.   Weeks or months.

Animals.   Eggs require 15 days to become infective. Worms mature three weeks after infection.

Clinical features
Humans.   Infection is usually subclinical. Visceral larva migrans affects children 1–4 years of age who may develop fever, asthmatic attacks, acute bronchiolitis, pneumonitis, nausea and vomiting, enlarged liver, spleen and lymph nodes, and possibly heart and CNS involvement. Ocular larva migrans usually affects older children in whom granulomatous nodules develop in the eye, with progressive loss of vision.

Animals.   It is usually subclinical, but massive prenatal infections can kill the puppies before 2–3 weeks of age.

Pathology
Humans and animals.   Larvae penetrate the mucosa of the small intestine and migrate to the liver and other tissues via blood vessels. Larvae bore through small vessels into surrounding tissues, producing granulomata around larvae or the shed surface components. Retinochoroiditis and peripheral retinitis and endophthalmitis may occur. Eosinophilia is prominent and persistent.

Special investigations
Humans.   Serological tests include ELISA and indirect fluorescent antibody tests. Demonstrate larvae in biopsy tissue.

Animals. Examine faeces for eggs.

Prognosis
Humans. The condition is usually benign. The ocular form can cause severe and progressive eye disease, even leading to blindness. The visceral form rarely causes CNS and heart involvement, which may be fatal.

Animals. It is benign in dogs and cats unless they become massively infected.

Prevention
Humans. Teach children good hygiene and prevent access to dog faeces. Keep dogs away from children's play areas. Cover sand-pits when not in use. Clean up faeces when exercising dogs in public parks.

Animals. Worm all dogs regularly.

Treatment
Humans. Diethylcarbamazine and thiabendazole are effective.

Animals. Worm all bitches and puppies.

Legislation
Humans and animals. None.

Toxoplasmosis/Congenital toxoplasmosis

A common and usually asymptomatic protozoal infection of humans. It occurs worldwide, but particularly in the tropics. Congenital infection in humans can lead to serious brain lesions.

The causative agent is *Toxoplasma gondii* (Protozoa). There is no vaccine.

Reservoir and mode of transmission
Definitive hosts are cats and wild felines of the genera Felis and Lynx. Cats are infected by eating raw meat, birds or

miçe containing parasite cysts. Faeces are a source of infection for other mammals and birds. Humans may be infected by eating raw or insufficiently cooked meat (mainly sheep, pigs, cattle or goats) and unwashed salad vegetables (*T. gondii* occurs in goat's milk, which is thus another source for human infection); or by ingestion of faecal oocysts from a cat's litter. Congenital infection of the fetus occurs when the human mother acquires primary infection in the second trimester of pregnancy.

Incubation period
Humans. Uncertain, but possibly 1–3 weeks.

Animals. Usually subclinical, but infected sheep frequently abort in the final month of pregnancy.

Clinical features
Humans. The acquired disease is usually asymptomatic, but there may be fever, headache, malaise, lymphadenopathy and cough of varying duration, and rarely myocarditis, encephalitis and pneumonitis. Severe cerebral infection can result from reactivation of latent infection in immunocompromised persons (e.g. AIDS patients). The congenital infection causes chronic retinitis, brain damage, hydrocephaly, microcephaly, enlarged liver and spleen, thrombocytopenia, rash and fever.

Animals. There are usually no signs of infection. In sheep it can cause severe economic loss from abortion towards the end of pregnancy. Congenitally infected lambs suffer incoordination, weakness and inability to feed. Sheep with encephalitis from toxoplasma infection walk in circles and suffer from muscle stiffness and prostration. Cats may show diarrhoea, hepatitis, myocarditis, myosytis, pneumonia and encephalitis if heavily infected, but are usually asymptomatic.

Pathology
Humans. Congenitally infected but surviving children show encephalitis with calcified foci in the brain, hydrocephalus and chorioretinitis. In immunosuppressed patients toxoplasmal cysts in the brain with encephalitis

may occur. Lymph nodes show characteristic irregular clusters of epithelioid cells with vesicular nuclei and eosinophilic cytoplasm. Infiltration of 'monocyte' cells produces distention of subcapsular and trabecular sinuses.

Animals. The characteristic lesions are toxoplasmal cysts in the brain with encephalitis. Grey foci of necrosis in the placental cotyledons are an important diagnostic sign.

Special investigations
Humans. Serological tests include the Sabin–Feldman dye test, indirect fluorescent antibody and ELISA tests. Isolate the organism by intraperitoneal inoculation of biopsy tissue into mice followed by brain histology. X-rays detect calcified plaques in the brain. There is characteristic histology of lymph node biopsies.

Animals. Isolate the organism in mice. Identify the oocysts microscopically.

Prognosis
Humans. Acquired infection is usually subclinical followed by solid immunity. Congenital infection leads to mental retardation, blindness, fits and hydrocephaly. In immunosuppressed patients there may be cerebral involvement which is often fatal.

Animals. Sheep abort but are immune thereafter.

Prevention
Humans. Pregnant women should avoid handling cat litter, or do so wearing gloves; and should wash hands after handling raw meat. Freezing may kill cysts in meat but thorough cooking is strongly recommended. Pregnant women should also avoid contact with lambing ewes. Apply strict laboratory safety procedures.

Animals. Prevent contamination of fodder by cat faeces.

Treatment
Humans. Anthelmintic treatment is usually not indicated and may be unsatisfactory. Severe allergic reactions may

follow killing of larvae, and steroids may be necessary to control these. Steroid treatment for eye involvement may control inflammation and oedema. Laser photocoagulation may be used.

Animals.   Inappropriate.

Legislation
Humans and animals.   None.

Trichinosis

[Trichiniasis, trichinellosis, trichinelliasis]

A severe roundworm infection acquired by eating under-cooked meat, especially pork. It occurs, sporadically and in small outbreaks, worldwide, but is probably absent from some countries such as the UK and Australia.

The causative agent is *Trichinella spiralis* (Nematoda). There is no vaccine.

Reservoir and mode of transmission
Reservoir hosts are carnivores, rats, pigs and bears. Humans are infected by ingesting encysted larvae in raw or undercooked meat (usually pork). Two large outbreaks in 1986 resulted from eating undercooked horse meat. Larvae penetrate the intestinal mucosa and develop to mature worms within 40 hours. Sexual reproduction leads to further larval stages. Within three days larvae may enter the circulation to encyst in muscle and other tissues.

Incubation period
Humans.   Variable, usually 10–14 days.

Animals.   Nearly always subclinical except in very heavy infection.

Clinical features
Humans.   Initially there is nausea, vomiting, diarrhoea, abdominal pain, muscle pains and weakness for a few days, followed by fever, oedema of the upper eyelids, retinal and subconjunctival haemorrhages, muscle swelling and tenderness for several weeks, and possibly myocarditis and

neurological signs. Dyspnoea due to pain in muscles.

Animals. Usually subclinical, but as for humans with very heavy infestation.

Pathology
Humans and animals. Larvae encyst in muscle and evoke a local inflammatory response. The cysts may become calcified. Eosinophilia is usual.

Special investigations
Humans and Animals. Serology. Identify larvae in muscle biopsy.

Prognosis
Humans. Illness usually lasts for 2–8 weeks with prolonged weakness. The fatality rate varies with the infecting load, but is about 5 per cent.

Animals. Usually subclinical, but very heavy infection can kill.

Prevention
Humans. Cooking (at 77°C or above) destroys the parasite. All pig meat should be properly inspected.

Animals. Prevent pigs gaining access to rats or uncooked offal.

Treatment
Humans. Thiabendazole coupled with supportive therapy to alleviate pain and inflammation.

Animals. Impracticable.

Legislation
Humans. The disease is notifiable in many countries, including the USA, Canada, New Zealand and several European countries.

Animals. Some countries require waste food to be heat-treated before being fed to pigs. Some require all pigmeat to be tested or frozen at – 25°C before its use as human food.

Tuberculosis (bovine)

[Bovine tuberculosis, consumption]

A potentially severe chronic bacterial disease usually acquired by drinking raw milk from infected cows.

The causative agent is *Mycobacterium bovis* (bacterium).

It occurs worldwide, but *M. bovis* has been almost eradicated from the cattle of several developed countries.

Reservoir and mode of transmission
Cattle are the natural reservoir of infection and transmission to humans is via consumption of raw milk. The organism poses a serious hazard to laboratory workers.

Incubation period
Humans.   Four weeks to several years.

Animals.   Variable.

Clinical features
Humans.   The primary lesion commonly causes enlarged cervical lymph nodes. This may be followed by extrapulmonary disease progressing over many months, with fever, weight loss, abdominal pain and tenderness, bone and joint lesions, genitourinary lesions, meningitis with neurological signs. Infection may be identical with respiratory tuberculosis.

Animals.   In cattle chronic disease remains subclinical for long periods but eventually leads to signs of chronic bronchopneumonia. Extensive destruction of lung tissue gives progressive respiratory distress and death. Swelling of the retropharyngeal lymph node may occur in calves. Milking cows may show a mild mastitis with progressive induration of the udder.

Pathology
Humans.   Caseating granulomatous lesions occur in tissues and lymph nodes, with calcification.

Animals. Granulomata form at the site of entry and spread to the local lymph nodes, which undergo caseation. Spread of infection throughout the body leads to miliary tuberculosis, but most lesions localize in the lung. Peritonitis may occur with a characteristic 'grape' type reaction. Infection of the udder gives progressive fibrosis with infection of milk.

Special investigations
Humans and animals. Skin test for reactivity to tuberculin. Also identify the mycobacterium by microscopy and culture of sputum, urine, cerebrospinal fluid or pus.

Prognosis
Humans. This is a slow, progressive disease leading to emaciation and death if untreated. Recurrences of infection may occur in later life.

Animals. Clinically affected animals and reactors to the tuberculin test are slaughtered.

Prevention
Humans. Heat-treat all milk. Identify and treat cases promptly. Ensure strict safety precautions in laboratories and immunize laboratory and health-care staff.

Animals. Total eradication of bovine tuberculosis in cattle has been virtually achieved in many countries by official test and slaughter policies.

Treatment
Humans. Antituberculous chemotherapy.

Animals. Not attempted.

Vaccination
Humans. BCG vaccine is given.

Animals. None.

Legislation
Humans.   The disease is notifiable is most countries.

Animals.   Some forms of tuberculosis in cattle are notifiable in certain countries. There are also voluntary or compulsory control schemes based on tuberculin testing with slaughter of reactors.

Tularaemia

[Francis' disease, deer-fly fever, rabbit fever, O'Haras disease]

A severe bacterial infection affecting rural populations, hunters and trappers, transmitted by contact with small wild mammals. The foci of infection are North America, the USSR, Japan and Europe.

The causative agent is *Francisella tularensis* (bacterium).

Reservoir and mode of transmission
The natural reservoirs are rabbits, hares, lemmings, rodents and other animals and birds, and their ticks. Transmission between animals and birds may be water-borne, air-borne, by ingestion of infected carcasses, by direct contact and by insect bite. Humans are usually infected by direct contact, or by inoculation accidents and insect bites. The organism poses a serious hazard to laboratory workers.

Incubation period
Humans.   1–10 days.

Animals.   Uncertain.

Clinical features
Humans.   The highly variable symptoms depend on the route of entry and the infecting dose. Usually there is sudden onset of fever, with headache and prostration which may persist for several weeks. In inoculation or insect bite transmission there will be an indolent ulcer with inflammation of local lymph nodes which then suppurate. Pneumonia may follow. A rash is common. Other forms of infection include primary pneumonia with pharyngitis, abscess formation, abdominal pain, vomiting and

diarrhoea; conjunctivitis and ulceration with pain in the eye, and lymphadenitis; chronic purulent lymphadenitis.

Animals. Clinical signs usually occur alongside heavy infestation with ticks, and include sudden high fever, anorexia and stiffness, eventually leading to prostration and death. In sheep, pregnant ewes may abort. Affected dogs have soft nodular swellings under the skin.

Pathology
Humans. Lesions include necrotic ulcer and reactive hyperplasia of lymph nodes and tonsils. Foci of necrosis occur in the liver, spleen and other organs. There may be bronchopneumonia.

Animals. Miliary foci of necrosis occur in the liver, spleen and lymph nodes. Severe lesions in the lung involve widespread consolidation with oedema and pleurisy.

Special investigations
Humans and animals. Isolate the organism by culture or inoculation of hamsters or guinea pigs. Serological tests include the fluorescent antibody test.

Prognosis
Humans. In the USA the untreated case fatality rate is about 5 per cent, but is lower in other countries. Survivors have a long convalescence of over 2–3 months.

Animals. Rodents and rabbits commonly die from septicaemia. Birds rarely die. Carnivores are rarely affected clinically.

Prevention
Humans. Avoid contamination of cuts and abrasions during skinning and evisceration of game carcasses. Cook meat thoroughly. Avoid tick bites. Control rodents. Immunize persons at high risk. Apply strict laboratory safety procedures.

Animals. Dip or spray sheep in enzootic areas.

Treatment
Humans.   Streptomycin is used. Penicillin is not effective.

Animals.   Broad-spectrum antibiotics, especially tetra-cyclines, are highly effective in sheep.

Vaccination
Humans.   Live attenuated vaccines are available in the USSR and the USA.

Animals.   No conclusively effective vaccine is available.

Legislation
Humans.   The disease is notifiable in several countries, including the USA and some European countries.

Animals.   None.

Vesicular stomatitis

[Sore mouth in cattle and horses]

A benign viral infection causing fever and vesicles in the mouth. It occurs in horses and cattle in many countries of the western hemisphere, but rarely affects humans exposed occupationally.

   The causative agents are the vesicular stomatitis viruses (Rhabdoviridae). There is no vaccine.

Reservoir and mode of transmission
The disease is not well understood. Horses, cattle and pigs are infected. It is probably spread by insect vectors and to humans in laboratory accidents.

Incubation period
Humans.   Uncertain, but probably 1–2 days.

Animals.   2–4 days.

Clinical features
Humans and animals.   Fever and influenza-like symptoms occur for a few days with vesicles in the mouth in some cases.

Pathology
Humans.   Uncertain.

Animals.   Vesicles occur on the feet and in the mouth.

Special investigations
Humans.   Serology. Isolate the virus from vesicles.

Animals.   Accurate identification is essential to distinguish from foot and mouth disease. The virus is identified in vesicle fluid by a complement fixation test. Animal inoculation is also used.

Prognosis
Humans.   It is a mild, self-limiting illness with full recovery in a few days.

Animals.   Recovery in one week.

Prevention
Humans.   Avoid contact with infected animals, and exercise care in the laboratory.

Animals.   Quarantine or prohibit importation of susceptible animals from affected countries.

Treatment
Humans.   Symptomatic therapy.

Animals.   None.

Legislation
Humans.   None.

Animals.   The disease is notifiable in horses, cattle and pigs in Tunisia, Sierra Leone, most of the American continent, Romania, Oman, Korea, Seychelles; in cattle and horses in Cyprus, New Zealand, Australia, Papua New Guinea; in cattle in Finland. In addition a slaughter policy applies to horses, cattle and pigs in the Falkland Islands, Finland, Greece and to horses and cattle in Czechoslovakia.

Wesselsbron disease

[Wesselsbron fever]

A benign, febrile, viral infection transmitted by mosquitoes from sheep and cattle. It occurs in South and West Africa.

The causative agent is the Wesselsbron virus (Togaviridae).

Reservoir and mode of transmission

Sheep and cattle serve as reservoirs. Mosquitoes transmit the infection to humans. Rodents and wildfowl may harbour the virus.

Incubation period

Humans.   2–4 days.

Animals.   1–4 days.

Clinical features

Humans.   Sudden onset of fever is followed by chills, headache, muscle and joint pains and sometimes a maculopapular rash. There may be encephalitis.

Animals.   Sheep are most susceptible and pregnant ewes abort and die. High mortality also occurs in neonatal lambs. Non-pregnant sheep suffer mild fever. Pregnant cattle also abort. Dogs show signs of encephalitis.

Pathology

Humans.   Not specific.

Animals.   Jaundice occurs with liver degeneration and foci of liver cell necrosis.

Special investigations

Humans and animals.   Isolate virus from blood; serology.

Prognosis

Humans.   It is usually a self-limiting infection, but muscle pains may persist.

Animals.   Slow recovery is usual. Newborn lambs commonly die.

Prevention
Humans.   Control mosquitoes and avoid their bites.

Animals.   Vaccinate sheep except for pregnant ewes.

Treatment
Humans.   Symptomatic therapy.

Animals.   None.

Vaccination
Humans.   None.

Animals.   An attenuated Wesselbron virus vaccine is available for sheep but it may induce abortion in pregnant ewes.

Legislation
Humans.   Acute encephalitis is notifiable in many countries, including the UK and the USA.

Animals.   None.

West Nile fever

A mosquito-borne viral infection occurring in Africa, Asia, the Middle East, France and Cyprus.
  The causative agent is the West Nile fever virus (Togaviridae). There is no vaccine.

Reservoir and mode of transmission
Many vertebrate hosts may harbour the virus. Wild birds are probably the most important reservoirs. Mosquitoes are vectors.

Incubation period
Humans.   3–6 days.

Animals.   Unknown.

Clinical features
Humans.   Sudden onset of fever is followed by headache, sore throat, muscle pains, lymphadenopathy, maculopapular rash for a few days and sometimes meningoencephalitis.

Animals.   Clinical signs are confined to horses but most cases are subclinical. Signs include meningoencephalitis.

Pathology
Humans and animals.   Meningoencephalitis including neuronal degeneration and perivascular cuffing with petaechial haemorrhages occur.

Special investigations
Humans.   Isolate the virus from blood by mouse inoculation. Serological tests include the haemagglutination, complement fixation and neutralization tests.

Animals.   Rarely undertaken, but as for humans.

Prognosis
Humans.   Usually self-limiting illness occurs with full recovery, but convalescence may be prolonged in adults.

Animals.   The case fatality rate of horses showing clinical signs is 25 per cent.

Prevention
Humans.   Control mosquitoes and avoid their bites.

Animals.   None.

Treatment
Humans.   Symptomatic therapy.

Animals.   None.

Legislation
Humans.   Acute encephalitis is notifiable in many countries, including the UK and the USA.

Animals.   None.

Yellow fever

[Black vomit]

A severe, febrile, mosquito-borne, viral disease leading to liver and kidney failure and death in many cases. It occurs as a zoonosis mainly in forest dwellers in the rain forest areas of northern South Africa, Central and South America.

The causative agent is the yellow fever virus (Togaviridae).

Reservoir and mode of transmission

The natural reservoirs of infection are forest monkeys, marmosets and humans. Transmission amongst monkeys by the bite of various species of mosquito in forests, and to people who enter or live near infected forests. There may also be an independent human/mosquito cycle in urban areas. The urban cycle has been almost eliminated by eradication of the mosquito vector, *Aedes aegypti*.

Incubation period

Humans.   3–6 days.

Animals.   Unknown.

Clinical features

Humans.   Most cases have fever, severe headache and backache, jaundice and albuminuria, followed by full recovery within a week, but in severe cases there is a second episode of fever, prostration, jaundice, renal failure and generalized haemorrhages.

Animals.   There is high fever and vomiting, with jaundice, oliguria and generalized haemorrhages in experimentally infected monkeys.

Pathology

Humans and animals.   Microglobular fatty degeneration of liver cells occurs with disruption of the hepatic lobule and necrosis of midzonal liver cells, producing so called

'Councilman' bodies. Degeneration and necrosis of the kidney tubules occurs. There are haemorrhages in tissues.

Special investigations

Humans.   Isolate the virus from blood in cell culture or in mice. Serological tests include haemagglutination inhibition and neutralization tests.

Animals.   Isolate the virus; serology.

Prognosis

Humans.   The case fatality rate is usually 5–10 per cent, but may be higher in epidemics.

Animals.   African primates rarely die as a result of experimental infection, whilst the disease is fatal in a few days in various American species.

Prevention

Humans.   Control mosquitoes and avoid their bites. Immunize exposed population and travellers.

Animals.   Eradicate mosquito vectors.

Treatment

Humans.   Symptomatic and supportive therapy.

Animals.   None.

Vaccination

Humans.   Live attenuated vaccine protects for at least ten years and is recommended for travellers to endemic areas and for the control of epidemics.

Animals.   None.

Legislation

Humans.   The disease is notifiable to WHO under International Health Regulations of 1969. An International Certificate of Vaccination is required from travellers by several African countries before admission.

Animals.   None.

Yersiniosis

[Pseudotuberculosis]

A usually self-limiting enteric bacterial infection which can be food-borne. It occurs worldwide, but particularly in Scandinavia and Canada.

The causative agents are *Yersinia pseudotuberculosis* and *Y. enterocolitica* (bacteria). There is no vaccine.

Reservoir and mode of transmission
Many species of wild and domestic animals and birds may be colonized. The main reservoir for human infection is not known. Food-borne infection from unpasteurized milk, cheese, raw pork and water have occurred, and person-to-person spread is possible.

Incubation period
Humans. 3–7 days.

Animals. Uncertain.

Clinical features
Humans. Acute onset of fever is followed by abdominal pain and diarrhoea for 1–3 weeks. Pharyngitis is a recently recognized relatively common symptom. Frequently the disease mimics appendicitis with right lower quadrant abdominal pain. Occasionally it is followed by arthritis and erythema nodosum.

Animals. Subacute clinical signs are common, with diarrhoea and weight loss, possibly with death in two weeks to three months. In sheep, abortions, epididymitis and orchitis occur with high mortality. In cattle abortion and pneumonia occur.

Pathology
Humans and animals. Acute inflammation of the terminal ileum with mesenteric lymphadenitis occurs. Sometimes abscesses develop in the liver, spleen and lungs.

Special investigations

Humans and animals.   Isolate the organism in faeces and blood and biopsy material, usually by cold enhancement.

Prognosis

Humans.   It is usually a self-limiting disease, but is occasionally associated with non-suppurative arthritis and skin lesions.

Animals.   Usually self-limiting, but there is a fatality rate of 5–7 per cent.

Prevention

Humans.   Control rodents and prevent contamination of food and water by rodents and birds. Pasteurize milk. Cook pork thoroughly. Personal hygiene is important (e.g. wash hands before eating and after handling animals).

Animals.   Impractical because of the wide range of animal hosts.

Treatment

Humans.   Illness is usually self-limiting, but antibiotics (e.g. tetracycline, chloramphenicol and gentamicin) may be indicated in severe infection.

Animals.   In outbreaks in poultry, cull those affected and treat the rest using antibiotics in feed or water.

Legislation

Humans.   The disease is notifiable specifically in Australia, and possibly if food-borne in other countries.

Animals.   None.

Zika fever

A poorly understood viral fever transmitted by mosquitoes from monkeys. It occurs in Africa.

The causative agent is the Zika virus (Togaviridae). There is no vaccine.

Reservoir and mode of transmission
The virus has been isolated from monkeys, mosquitoes and humans. Serological studies suggest widespread infection. Transmission to humans is probably from mosquito bites and laboratory accidents.

Incubation period
Humans and animals.   Uncertain.

Clinical features
Humans. There is fever, malaise and sometimes a maculopapular rash for a few days.

Animals. Uncertain.

Pathology
Humans. Not specific.

Animals. Uncertain.

Special investigations
Humans and animals. Isolate the virus from blood by inoculation of suckling mice. Serological tests include haemagglutination and neutralization tests.

Prognosis
Humans. It is usually a self-limiting illness.

Animals. Uncertain.

Prevention
Humans. Control mosquitoes and avoid mosquito bites.

Animals. None.

Treatment
Humans. Symptomatic.

Animals. None.

Legislation
Humans and animals. None.

Definitions of some terms used in this text

Animal products
Any useful substance derived from animals, including milk, eggs, meat, offal, glandular extracts, wool, hides, hair, tallow, gelatine, glue, protein and bone meals used for animal feeds or fertilizers.

Carrier
Used in this text in the sense of 'biological' carrier: an animal or person clinically well but with an infection (q.v.), and who may from time to time excrete the infectious agent.

Contagious
A disease which may be transmitted by contact, either direct or indirect, with other infected individuals.

Contact
A 'contact' is a person or animal that has been in contact with an infected individual or contaminated environment.

Contamination
The presence of an infectious agent on the body surface or on an inanimate object.

Cleansing
Removal of infective material by washing, hosing, scrubbing, usually using soaps and detergents and an essential preliminary to disinfection (q.v.).

Disinfection
Physical or chemical removal of infectious agents from a contaminated place or object or so treating them that they are killed or no longer infective. Physical disinfection includes mechanical removal of infectious agents or exposing them to sunlight, desiccation and high temperatures, and burying infected carcasses. Chemical disinfectants include coal tar derivatives, formaldehyde, halogens, quaternary ammonium compounds, hot washing soda, ammonia, aqueous solution of alcohol. Leaving premises empty for a period after an outbreak of contagious disease is a common and useful sequel to cleansing and disinfection.

Endemic
Disease or infection usually present in the human population within a given geographic area.

Epidemic
Unusual increase in occurrence of a disease in a human population.

Enzootic
Disease or infection usually present in an animal population within a given geographical area.

Epizootic
Unusual increase in occurrence of a disease in an animal population.

Eradication
Systematic, state-controlled measures to reduce the prevalence of a disease in an animal or human population in a defined geographical area, the final aim being complete elimination of that infection. Often attempted by a test and slaughter policy (q.v.) in animals.

Exposure
Being in a situation in which contact with an infectious agent is likely.

Fumigation
Any process by which living organisms, especially viruses, bacteria, arthropods and rodents, are killed by use of disinfectants or poisons in gaseous or aerosol form.

Host
A vertebrate or invertebrate in which an infectious agent lives under natural conditions. An accidental host is a person or animal which is not part of a natural disease cycle and does not usually transmit the infection. An intermediate host is a vertebrate or invertebrate in which a parasite completes an essential, asexual part of its life-cycle. A final host is usually a vertebrate in which a parasite completes the sexual part of its life-cycle.

Incidence
The rate of occurrence of a disease in a population.

Incubation period
The time interval between contact with an infectious agent and the appearance of the first sign or symptom.

Infection
The entry into and development or multiplication of an infectious agent in the body. In latent infection an inapparent (asymptomatic, subclinical) infection is capable of becoming overt disease under certain circumstances (e.g. lowering of the host's resistance). Infectious agents are living organisms (bacteria, rickettsias, chlamydias, viruses, protozoa, helminths, fungi) capable of producing infectious disease (clinical manifestations of infection).

Isolation
Separation of infected persons or animals from members of the same or other susceptible species during the period of communicability. Also the act of demonstrating the presence of an infectious agent by growing it in pure culture in the laboratory.

Mode of transmission
Used in this text to summarize those factors which lead to transmission of infection or disease from one host to

another, and includes aspects of the infectious agent's life-cycle, reservoir, intermediate and final hosts, the agent's resistance to environmental factors and the route of infection (e.g. ingestion, inhalation, inoculation).

Notifiable disease
A disease the presence or suspicion of which is reportable by law to a regulatory authority so that appropriate control measures may be applied.

Prevalence
The number of individuals affected by a disease at a particular time expressed as a proportion of the population.

Pandemic
An epidemic (q.v.) affecting several countries or continents.

Panzootic
An epizootic (q.v.) affecting several countries or continents.

Quarantine
Restriction of activities to prevent the spread of infection of a person who has been exposed to infection and may therefore be infectious during its incubation period; or isolation of animals so exposed from susceptible animals of the same or other species.

Reservoir
Vertebrate or invertebrate animal, plant, soil or substance in which an infectious agent (q.v.) normally lives and multiplies, on which it depends for its survival and from which it can be transmitted to a host (q.v.).

Sporadic
Used in this text to indicate a case of a disease, which may be endemic, apparently unconnected with an outbreak.

Outbreak
Two or more connected cases of a disease within a human population or amongst the same animal species.

Slaughter policy
Applied by a state which has taken legal powers to slaughter animals affected by a particular disease and, usually, their contacts (q.v.).

Vehicle of infection
A non-living thing which transports an infectious agent to a human or animal.

Vector
A living organism which transmits disease from host to host. Control methods include: destruction of vectors and elimination of their breeding places by burning and cultivation of scrub land, filling ponds and draining marshes; removal of vectors' food supply by slaughter or movement control of game; application of insecticides by dip or spray to animals and by spray to houses and around villages or camps. Vermin are controlled by poison baits and by making buildings vermin-proof.

Zoonoses
Infections transmissible under natural conditions between vertebrate animals and humans.

Index